# PROGRESSIVE EXERCISE THERAPY

## IN REHABILITATION AND PHYSICAL EDUCATION

BY

John H. C. Colson FCSP FSRG DipTRG DipCOT

*Remedial Therapy Representative, NHS Health Advisory Service. Formerly Director of Rehabilitation and Principal, School of Remedial Gymnastics and Recreational Therapy, Pinderfields General Hospital*
and

Frank W. Collison MSRG

*Head Remedial Gymnast and Clinical Supervisor, Rehabilitation Department, Pinderfields General Hospital. Formerly Head Remedial Gymnast, Orsett Hospital*

FOURTH EDITION

WRIGHT · PSG

BRISTOL · LONDON · BOSTON
1983

*Published by:* John Wright & Sons Ltd, 823–825 Bath Road, Bristol BS4 5NU,
England
John Wright PSG Inc., 545 Great Road, Littleton,
Massachusetts 01460, USA.

*First edition* 1958
*Japanese edition* 1966
*Second edition* 1969
*Spanish edition* 1974
*Third edition* 1975
*Dutch edition* 1981
*Fourth edition* 1983

*British Library Cataloguing in Publication Data*

Colson, John H. C.
    Progressive exercise therapy in rehabilitation
    and physical education.
    1. Exercise therapy
    I. Title    II. Collison, Frank W.
    615.8′24    RM725

ISBN 0 7236 0665 X

Library of Congress Catalog Card Number: 82-50781

*Printed in Great Britain by*
John Wright & Sons (Printing) Ltd, at The Stonebridge Press, Bristol BS4 5NU

*The Wise, for Cure, on Exercise depend.* DRYDEN.

# PREFACE

The first edition of this book appeared in 1958. Its main aim was to emphasize the importance of progression in exercise therapy and to provide a comprehensive collection of free exercises for all parts of the body, graded and progressed (as the original preface had it) in strength and mobility from the simplest to the most strenuous movement.

Since that time two other editions have appeared and the book has been translated into Japanese, Spanish and Dutch. From comments received from students and therapists it is clear that the practical slant of the book has been appreciated. Indeed, it has been heartening to receive so many letters from different countries offering criticism, encouragement and suggestions for future editions.

This new edition of *Progressive Exercise Therapy*, written in collaboration with my friend and former colleague, Frank Collison, has not only been completely revised, but expanded to include new sections on assisted and resisted exercises, functional movement, progressive circuit training and exercises to music. In addition, the section devoted to the exercise therapy of various clinical conditions (which illustrates the way in which the exercise vocabulary may be used when planning treatment programmes) has been rewritten to bring it into line with modern practice. Running the risk of criticism we have included a chapter on the re-educational measures which may be used in the treatment of total hip replacement when the low friction Charnley prosthesis is employed.

Unfortunately, the addition of so much new material has meant the deletion of the sections on recreational therapy in the treatment of the mentally handicapped and the mentally ill, which appeared in the previous edition. Limitation of space has also meant that it has not been possible to include any reference to the important role played by neurophysiological techniques in modern exercise therapy.

We owe much to the late John M. P. Clark, Emeritus Professor of Orthopaedic Surgery, University of Leeds, not only for his constant encouragement and advice but for his truly superb teaching at ward rounds and clinics. For 'Pasco' exercise therapy was the straight and narrow path to recovery after injury or disease, and progression the keynote of success.

Our sincere thanks are due to the surgeons who have given us so much practical help. Mr J. F. Patrick FRCS, Mr A. E. Rainey FRCS, and Mr C. Robertson FRCS, of the Orthopaedic Department, Pinderfields General Hospital, Wakefield, Yorkshire, were always willing to guide us on technical matters during the preparation of the chapters on orthopaedic procedures. Mr C. Denley Clark FRCS and Mr G. Bird FRCS gave us generous support when we were involved in the revision of the section on the use of exercise therapy after abdominal surgery.

It is also a great pleasure to acknowledge the help given by the nursing staff of the orthopaedic and general surgical wards at Pinderfields General Hospital. Their appreciation of the value of early movement, and their detailed understanding of modern surgical techniques and equipment, have made for the closest cooperation during practical sessions of exercise therapy.

Our grateful thanks are due also to Mr John V. Gough MCSP DipTP, for his advice and help when investigating the use of the myometer in recording muscle strength. It is also a great pleasure to acknowledge the outstanding help given by Mr Robbie Blake MCSP DipTP during the many months of preparing the revised text of this book. He has listened, commented and criticized in a most useful and constructive way.

The staff of the Wakefield and District Postgraduate Medical Centre gave us valuable help with the checking of references and the compiling of the bibliography; they also made available the resources of their information service. We are grateful to the team concerned and in particular to Mrs Cecily A. Miller, BA DipLib ALA, head of information services.

Finally, we must thank our Editor, Dr Sue Passmore, for her interest in the book and her enthusiasm for the subject matter. Our thanks must also be extended to our publishers, John Wright & Sons, for their support and cooperation over many years.

John Colson
Frank Collison

# CONTENTS

# PART 1

# SPECIFIC EXERCISE THERAPY

# 1. Introductory

Specific or local exercises consist of active movements that are designed to restore function. General exercises, on the other hand, are those that provide movement for the body as a whole.

Specific exercises are used to strengthen particular muscle groups, mobilize certain joints or re-educate neuromuscular coordination, and are of great value in the treatment of injuries and disorders of the locomotor system where certain muscle groups and joints are affected and the rest are comparatively normal, e.g. in fractures and other bone and joint injuries, orthopaedic conditions, thoracic diseases and postoperative abdominal conditions.

Specific exercises are not sufficient in themselves to bring about perfect functional recovery, however, for muscles and joints were never intended by nature to act as individualists. For the best results specific exercises must be combined with general exercises, so as to coordinate the movements of the affected part with the rest of the locomotor system. It is also often necessary to combine treatment by exercises with passive therapy, occupational therapy and various recreational activities—games, swimming, walking and cycling.

## TYPES OF SPECIFIC EXERCISES

Specific exercises consist of *free* movements, *assisted* movements and *resisted* movements. The movements, and the various techniques used to achieve progression, are considered in detail in the next three chapters.

## BASIC PRINCIPLES OF SPECIFIC EXERCISES

All types of specific exercises must conform to certain basic principles:

1. They must be performed in a smooth and rhythmical manner, so that they do not subject muscles and joints to sudden unexpected stresses and strains.

2. They must be based on sound starting positions.

3. They must provide smooth progression from the stage of extreme weakness to the stage of full use against the stresses of normal working conditions.

In addition, all exercises that aim to strengthen weak muscles should provide as wide a range of movement as possible.

## Principle of Rhythm

Muscular contraction must be followed by relaxation, and the relaxation period must be complete and long enough to allow normal circulatory conditions to be restored. This principle applies particularly to exercises which are used to redevelop weak muscles after trauma or disuse. It is based on the fact that the efficiency of a muscle depends largely on the condition of its local circulation. If this is good, the breakdown products of contraction are quickly carried away; if it is poor, the products tend to accumulate and produce early fatigue.

To conform to the principle of rhythm in practice the therapist must give as much emphasis to the relaxation period at the end of an exercise as to the actual muscle work itself. Thus, in using an exercise like *Fixed prone lying; Trunk bending backwards with Arm turning outwards (Fig.* 1a, p. 8), to strengthen the extensor muscles of the thoracolumbar spine, the following type of coaching might be used.

'Bend back the head—turn out the arms so that the palms face forward—lift the chest from the floor as far as you can . . . A little more . . . Now "hold" the position for a moment . . . Lower the trunk down carefully; let the arms turn in . . . Now turn the head and flop out completely. Let everything go. . . .' After a few seconds' pause the exercise is repeated.

It is worth comparing this technique with that often used for the same type of exercise. 'Lift—! Hold the position! Lower . . . Rest . . . Lift—!' The instructions for relaxation and the restarting of the exercise almost merge into one another and completely negate the principle of rhythm.

## Sound Starting Position

The starting position from which each exercise is performed should facilitate the work of the muscles, and be suitable for the particular phase of recovery reached by the patient.

### Strengthening and Mobilizing

To strengthen weak muscles or to mobilize stiff joints the starting positions of the exercises should be as steady as possible, so as to give the working muscles a firm origin from which to work. The larger the base of support the steadier will be the position of the body. For example, stride standing is steadier than standing, sitting steadier than stride standing and lying a steadier position than sitting. The nearer the centre of gravity to the base of support, the steadier is the position.

In some instances additional stability is achieved by arranging for the base to be enlarged in the direction of the movement. For example, walk-forwards standing is a steadier position than stride standing for exercises in which the arms are moved in the sagittal plane, because the movements of the arms cause the centre of gravity of the body to be constantly shifted forwards and backwards. This is particularly evident when vigorous wide range arm movements are performed, such as *Arm swinging forwards and forwards-upwards*. In stride standing the compensatory balancing required is achieved not only by essential small movements of the ankle joints but very often by unnecessary movements in the lumbar spine, with the head and pelvis moving forwards and backwards alternately.

*Developing Coordination*
In developing neuromuscular coordination the starting position should be chosen so as gradually to increase the difficulty of maintaining the balance, e.g. toe standing and standing with one knee raised forwards.

## Principle of Progression
The method of progression used depends on whether an exercise is designed to redevelop strength, restore mobility or redevelop neuromuscular coordination. One method of progression, however, is common to all types of exercises: progression in time. That is, performing the exercise for increasing periods of time.

## Wide Range Movements
Except in the early phase of recovery when the muscles are very weak, all exercises which aim at strengthening muscles should provide as wide a range of movement as possible, and each movement should be taken to its limit. In this way it is more likely that all the fibres of the muscle responsible for the movement will be exercised normally. This is important, because it appears from the action of certain muscles that individual groups of muscle fibres are responsible for particular ranges of movement. In other words, exercising a muscle in part of its range of movement does not necessarily mean that all its fibres will be brought into action.

The classic example of this is the vastus medialis muscle. The lower fibres 'contract particularly during the terminal phase of extension of the knee joint to retain the patella in its groove on the patellar surface of the femur . . .' (Williams and Warwick, 1980). Therefore, failure to extend the knee to its full extent when exercising the quadriceps femoris muscle group means that although the vastus lateralis and rectus femoris sections are exercised fully the vastus medialis is inadequately exercised. *See also* p. 23.

## REFERENCE

Williams P. L. and Warwick R. (1980) *Gray's Anatomy*, 36th ed. London, Churchill Livingstone.

# 2. Free exercises

Free exercises are performed by the patient without external assistance or resistance (beyond that exerted by gravity), although in some instances they are controlled by gymnastic apparatus. They consist of simple, everyday functional movements and gymnastic exercises drawn from the main systems of physical education.

Free movements are not confined to any one phase of recovery, although the gymnastic type of movement is reserved more especially for the intermediate and final phases. In general, they are employed more often than any other form of remedial exercises. This is because they make the patient rely on his own efforts, are particularly suitable for group and class work, and do not require specialized equipment beyond the normal type of gymnasium apparatus.

## 1. PROGRESSION IN STRENGTH

Progression in strength is of great importance in the treatment of injury and disease, because without muscle strength range of movement is relatively useless. On the other hand, strength without range is frequently compatible with full function under the stresses imposed by heavy occupations.

### Methods of Progression

There are seven main methods of progressing the strength of free exercises:

1. By increasing the length of the weight arm of the lever, i.e. arranging the movement so that the centre of gravity of the moving part is further away from the moving joint than before. For example, *Trunk bending backwards* from *fixed prone lying* is harder work for the extensors of the thoracolumbar spine and hips when the arms are placed in *neck rest* than when they are by the sides (cf. *Fig.* 1*a* and *b*). The exercise is made more difficult if the arms are held in *stretch* position (*Fig.* 1*c*).

A modification of this type of progression is used in strengthening the spinal rotator muscles in the pelvic rotation exercise shown in *Fig.* 2. In *Fig.* 2*a* (*Leg lowering sideways* from *half-crook half-leg lift lying*) the raised leg acts as a single lever. In *Fig.* 2*b* (*slow Leg swinging from side to side* from *vertical leg*

7

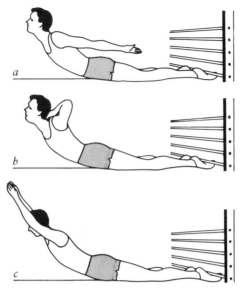

Fig. 1. Progression in strength: increasing the length of the weight arm of the lever.

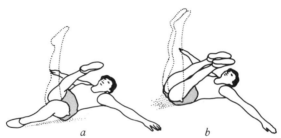

Fig. 2. Progression in strength: rotator muscles of thoracic spine. The combined weight of the two-leg lever in *b* is a strong progression on the single-leg lever of *a*.

*lift lying*) the combined weight of the two levers forms a strong progression on the single-lever system of the first exercise.

It should be noted that the pelvic rotation exercise, *Knee swinging from side to side* from *yard crook lying* (*Fig.* 128, p. 100), is basically a mobility exercise and is therefore not included in this group.

2. By 'cutting out' the help given to the prime mover muscles by accessory muscles. For example, *Lying; high Leg raising to touch the floor overhead with the toes* is harder work for the abdominal muscles when the arms are in *reach* (*Fig.* 3*b*) or *stretch* position than when they are by the sides (*Fig.* 3*a*). In the latter position the accessory flexor muscles of the thoracolumbar spine (latissimus dorsi, teres major and pectoralis major) come into action to assist the

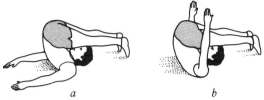

*Fig.* 3. Progression in strength: eliminating the help given to the abdominal muscles by the accessory flexor muscles of the thoracolumbar spine.

abdominals. They work strongly in inner range, and the first two muscle groups produce extension of the shoulder joint in addition to spinal flexion. Extension is associated, after some 15°, with shoulder girdle movement.

In general, the most difficult starting position for this exercise is lying with the arms stretched sideways in *yard* position. This is because the position of the arms makes it difficult for the performer to pivot at the thoracocervical junction, and he has to use his abdominal muscles strongly in an attempt to bring about additional flexion of the thoracolumbar spine.

3. By increasing the range of movement. For example, *spanning* performed from angle-hanging (*Fig.* 4*b*) is harder work than when it is performed from the *high reach grasp crook lying* position (*Fig.* 4*a*). The exercise is made more difficult still when it is performed from *stretch grasp back support long sitting* (*Fig.* 4*c*).

4. By the addition of subsidiary movements to an exercise, so as to increase the work of the main muscle group. For example, *Prone lying; Trunk bending*

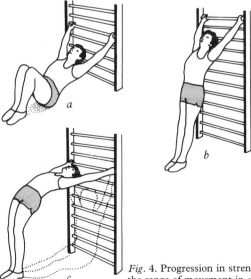

*Fig.* 4. Progression in strength: increasing the range of movement in *spanning*.

*backwards with Arm turning outwards and single Leg raising backwards* (*Fig.* 5) is harder work for the extensors of the thoracolumbar spine than the same exercise without leg movements. Raising both legs backwards at the same time (instead of one leg in turn) makes the exercise more difficult still.

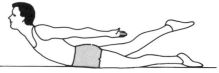

*Fig.* 5. Progression in strength: subsidiary movements are added to the exercise to increase the work of the main muscle group.

5. By using first static and then dynamic muscle work. For example, (*a*) *Half lying; single Quadriceps contractions*, and (*b*) *Half lying* (*thighs supported by folded pillow or shaped wooden block, with knees flexed to about 30°*); *single Knee stretching*.

6. By altering the rhythm of the movement. Slow, controlled movements require more effort from the muscles than the same movements performed at a quicker rate.

7. By altering the effect of gravity on the moving part, i.e. arranging for the movement to be performed with gravity stresses eliminated, and later against the resistance of gravity. Thus, in strengthening the rotators of the thoracic spine: (*a*) *Stride sitting; Trunk turning*, and (*b*) *Stride lying; Trunk turning with single Arm carrying across the chest* (*Fig.* 129, p. 101).

## 2. PROGRESSION IN RANGE

From the viewpoint of function, range of movement is undoubtedly secondary in importance to muscle strength. In the restoration of stiff joints after trauma, however, very little headway would be made without employing specific mobility exercises.

### Methods of Progression

There are three main methods of progressing the range of free mobility exercises:

1. By altering the rhythm of the movement. For example, rhythmical swingings are used in place of slow movements.

2. By adding a series of small rhythmical pressing movements to the end of the main movement, e.g. *Stride standing; Trunk bending from side to side with rhythmical pressing to three counts in position.*

3. By introducing prolonged tension movements. For example, in increasing the range of flexion of a stiff knee joint, the patient lies on his back with the knee and hip joints of the affected limb flexed as much as possible without producing pain. He attempts to relax the quadriceps femoris muscle completely, so as to allow the lower leg to hang as a dead weight from the knee. He then contracts the hamstring muscles strongly until the knee is flexed to the limit of pain, 'holds' the position for several seconds, and then allows the hamstrings to relax slowly. This procedure is repeated several times before the knee joint is extended.

### 3. PROGRESSION IN COORDINATION

The main methods of progression may be divided into those that are applicable to all parts of the body, and those that are chiefly applicable to the lower limbs and trunk.

### General Methods of Progression

1. Giving movements of the large joints first, and movements of the smaller joints later, e.g. shoulder movements require less coordination than finger movements.

2. Increasing the precision with which a controlled movement is performed.

3. Combining movements of different joints, e.g. *Knee full bending with Arm raising sideways*. An extension of this form of progression consists of performing asymmetrical movements, e.g. *opposite Arm swinging sideways and forwards*.

### Methods Applicable to Lower Limbs and Trunk

1. Diminishing the size of the accustomed base of support, so that the maintenance of balance becomes a matter of concentrated attention. Generally this is done by (a) bringing the feet together (*close standing*); (b) raising the heels from the floor (*toe standing*); (c) raising one foot from the floor, e.g. *Standing; single Knee raising*; and (d) standing or walking on a narrow surface such as a balance bench rib or beam.

2. Increasing the difficulties of assuming or maintaining the balance position by (a) placing the arms in a higher positon (e.g. *stretch*), so as to raise the centre of gravity of the body; (b) moving the free joints, and so disturbing the balance, e.g. *Balance half standing (beam)*; *single Knee raising with Arm raising sideways-upwards*; and (c) increasing the height of the apparatus used, which (because of psychological factors) disturbs the equilibrium considerably (*Fig. 6*).

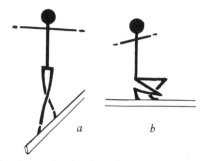

*Fig.* 6. Progression in coordination: increasing the difficulty of maintaining the balance position by raising the height of the apparatus used.

## Rhythmical Hopping and Skipping

Rhythmical hopping and skipping exercises which demand considerable balance are extremely useful in promoting coordination. For example: (*a*) *Hopping with alternate Toe placing forwards and sideways (Fig.* 7); (*b*) *Running*

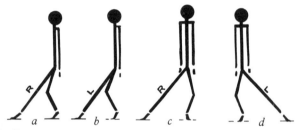

*Fig.* 7. Progression in coordination: Hopping with alternate Toe placing forwards and sideways.

*on the spot with high Knee raising, stopping in position on one leg at a given command;* (*c*) *Skipping: skip jump with rebound, moving forwards, backwards, right and left, 6 counts in each direction;* and (*d*) *Skipping: hopping with a rebound and alternate Knee stretching (Fig.* 8).

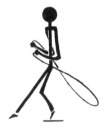

*Fig.* 8. Progression in coordination: Skipping—hopping with a rebound and alternate Knee stretching.

# 3. Assisted exercises

## 1. ASSISTED ACTIVE EXERCISES

Assisted active exercises are those performed by the patient with the assistance of the therapist or some outside force, such as a cord and pulley or weight-and-pulley circuit. They are used when the muscles acting on one of the body levers are too weak to bring about movement or to control it adequately. They are also used in the restoration of mobility.

The assistance or external force employed is applied in the direction of the muscle action. It should be sufficient to give adequate help to the working muscles, but must not be allowed to exceed this level or a passive movement will result.

Whatever type of assistance is used the underlying objective must be to secure the best possible working conditions for the weak muscles and to eliminate any muscle work other than that which is necessary to achieve the desired movement. Thus the moving part must be supported fully throughout the movement, and the body stabilized by a sound starting position.

Four examples of different types of assisted active movements are given here:

(a) *Lying; flexion of the Hip and Knee with therapist's assistance (Fig. 9).*

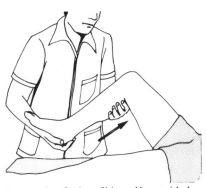

*Fig.* 9. Assisted active exercise: flexion of hip and knee with therapist's assistance.

(b) *Sitting (chair); elevation of the Arm through abduction with cord and pulley circuit (Fig. 10).*

13

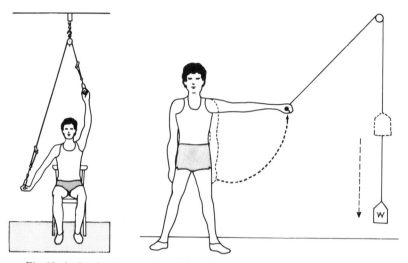

*Fig.* 10. Assisted active exercise with cord and pulley circuit: elevation of arm through abduction.

*Fig.* 11. Assisted active exercise with weight-and-pulley circuit: abduction of shoulder joint.

(c) *Stride standing; assisted abduction of the Shoulder joint with weight-and-pulley circuit* (*Fig.* 11).

(d) *Sitting on stool or bench in pool (the water level with the top of the shoulders); buoyancy-assisted abduction of the Shoulder joint* (*Fig.* 12).

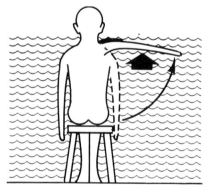

*Fig.* 12. Buoyancy-assisted abduction of shoulder joint. (Illustration reproduced from 'Basic hydrotherapy', *Physiotherapy* (1981), **67**, 258–262, by kind permission of the author, Anne Golland MCSP, and the Editor of the Journal.)

*Progression*

As the strength of the muscles improves the degree of assistance provided must be gradually diminished.

## 2. AUTO-ASSISTED ACTIVE (TENSION) EXERCISES

Auto-assisted active (tension) exercises are used to restore the mobility of some of the larger joints—in particular, the knee and shoulder—where stiffness is due to thickenings and adhesions within the joints and their capsules. They are only employed in the intermediate and late phases of recovery and are reserved for joints which are free from effusion. They are contraindicated in the treatment of elbow injuries.

The exercises resemble assisted active movements carried out with a cord and pulley circuit, but include a stressing or tension element which is controlled entirely by the patient. They are extremely valuable, but need careful teaching and supervision.

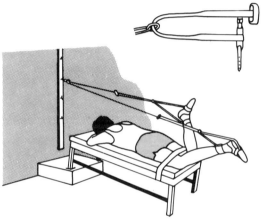

*Fig.* 13. Auto-assisted active (tension) exercise: flexion of the knee joint. The circuit may be used to restore the range of flexion from 0 to 130°. In practice it has been found best to use the combined circuits shown in *Fig.* 14 to restore the first 40–60° of flexion. Note the simple device used to raise the head end of the plinth and prevent it moving forwards when the patient is exercising, and the series of hooks arranged on a wall-mounted upright: they allow easy adjustment of the circuit's angle of pull. The foot and ankle straps shown are made from soft leather. Each set consists of a circular foot cuff and adjustable ankle strap. The cuff and strap are connected by a leather 'cord' which carries a free-moving galvanized ring. The ends of the circuit cord are looped through these rings.

*Fig.* 13 shows an auto-assisted active (tension) circuit arranged to assist flexion of the knee. *Fig.* 14 demonstrates the use of combined weight-and-pulley and cord and pulley circuits in the restoration of knee flexion. The simple cord and pulley circuit shown in *Fig.* 10 can be used to bring about auto-assisted active (tension) movements of the shoulder joint.

*Exercise Technique*

In performing an auto-assisted active (tension) exercise the patient should

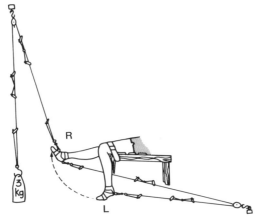

*Fig.* 14. Auto-assisted active flexion of the knee joint: combined cord and pulley and weight-and-pulley circuits. The combined circuits offer a smooth and effective means of restoring the first 60° of flexion. The resistance weight used should be sufficient to counterbalance the lower leg. From the starting position demonstrated the patient flexes the stiff knee joint (R), simultaneously extending the sound knee joint (L). The movements must be synchronized so that the cord and pulley circuit is kept under even tension throughout. When the stiff joint reaches the point when assistance is required the patient reinforces the prime mover muscles by a small movement of extension of the sound joint— which exerts increased tension on the cord and pulley circuit. After 'holding' the final position for a moment the patient allows the resistance weight to extend the stiff knee joint, and slackens off the extensor muscles of the sound knee so that it returns to its original starting position.

adjust the length of the circuit cord, so that it is reasonably taut and therefore responsive to movement. He then moves the affected limb in the required direction, simultaneously moving the other limb in the opposite direction so as to keep the cord taut.

When the affected limb enters the stiff painless zone of movement (*see below*) and reaches the point when assistance is required, the patient endeavours to take the movement still further with the prime mover muscles, and at the same time reinforces them by further tension on the cord with the sound limb. On reaching the painful limit he 'holds' the position for a moment, and then returns the limbs to their starting position by a reversal of the previous movements. Throughout, the exercise should be performed smoothly and fairly slowly.

*Zones of Movement*

With regard to the tension aspect of the exercises it is worth noting that there are three ranges or zones of movement in a stiff joint: (*a*) a range of free and painless movement, which is generally the largest; (*b*) a range of stiffness with little or no pain; and (c) a range of stiffness and pain. Beyond this range there is complete loss of movement.

In performing auto-assisted active (tension) movements the patient should work in the inner part of the first range, and through the second range, which is usually small. He should avoid the third range, for it is this that sets up reactions. Indeed, exercising in this zone is the equivalent of forcible stretching. Evidence of over-treatment will be found in swelling and increasing pain, and in stationary or diminishing movement.

## 3. SUSPENSION AND SUPPORTED EXERCISES

Suspension and supported exercises are widely used in the early redevelopment of weak muscles and the restoration of mobility. In general, they offer indirect assistance to the working muscles by freeing them of frictional and gravity stresses.

### Suspension Exercises

In suspension exercises the parts of the body to be exercised are supported by canvas slings attached by adjustable-length cords to an overhead point or points, so that a certain degree of elevation is achieved (*see Figs.* 15 and 16). In this way the body is relieved of the frictional stresses encountered when movement is attempted on a horizontal supporting surface, such as a bed or plinth. Metal or wooden runners fitted to the cords ensure easy adjustment of the suspension unit.

#### Axial Fixation

The overhead attachment point of the cords is positioned immediately above the joint to be exercised. When movement is initiated it occurs throughout the horizontal plane, the prime mover muscles being indirectly assisted as the part is gravity-free and therefore weightless. This allows considerable scope for varying the type of activity used—from rhythmical swinging movements, to assist mobility and promote the circulation in the region of the joint, to slow controlled movements to increase muscle strength. *Fig.* 15 shows the method of arranging axial fixation to promote abduction and adduction movements of the hip.

#### Co-axial Fixation

Axial fixation can be modified to produce some degree of resistance or assistance for individual muscle groups. The overhead fixation point of the cords is then moved to one side of the joint. For example, if the abductor muscles of the hip are to be resisted, the fixation point is sited over the

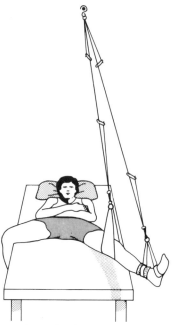

*Fig.* 15. Suspension exercise: axial fixation used to promote abduction and adduction movements of the hip joint. The overhead attachment point of the suspension cords is positioned immediately above the joint.

adductors of the joint; automatically, this causes the lower limb to assume an adducted position when at rest. When the abductors are activated the lower limb rises slightly into abduction (in the form of a pendular movement) with gravity offering resistance.

Gravity will also return the limb to the adducted position passively if the abductors are relaxed completely; this can be used as an early form of assisted movement for the adductors. Conversely, if the return movement is controlled actively the abductors will work excentrically against gravity.

### Vertical Fixation

The overhead fixation point of the cord and sling unit is positioned directly over the centre of gravity of the part to be supported, i.e. over the junction of the upper and middle one-thirds.

Vertical suspension has a stabilizing effect on the part supported; movement is restricted to small-range pendular movements. Because of this, vertical fixation is used to give support rather than to encourage movement (*Fig.* 16). It is sometimes employed as a means of achieving either local or general relaxation; short tension springs are incorporated into the overhead aspect of the cord and sling unit or units to provide 'buoyancy'.

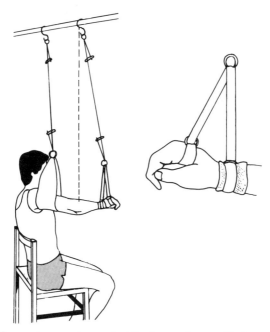

*Fig.* 16. Suspension exercise: vertical fixation used to provide firm support for the upper arm, while axial suspension promotes movement of the elbow joint. The overhead attachment point of the axial suspension unit is sited directly over the joint. *Inset*: radial aspect of hand and wrist, showing felt cuff used to protect soft tissues from pressure of self-locking sling.

## Suspension Equipment

In the physiotherapy department overhead fixation points for suspension work are usually provided by a rectangular-shaped grill of strong 5 cm metal mesh, which is sited over a plinth and roughly approximates to its surface area. The grill is securely fastened to the ceiling joists, with a 1·5 m clearance between plinth top and mesh.

Where ceiling fixation is not possible a free-standing tubular steel suspension frame (originated by the late Mrs O. F. Guthrie-Smith) can be used in conjunction with a plinth to provide the necessary suspension points.

In the ward situation the adjustable overhead cross-bars of the orthopaedic framework of a modern variable-height bed are often used to provide fixation points. On occasions, too, the hook end of a 'monkey pole', securely fastened to the bed-head, serves as a useful fixation point. Unfortunately, both adaptations have the disadvantage of reducing the length of the suspension cords, which restricts the range of movement achieved by the patient.

A comprehensive account of all forms of suspension movement, including techniques for the trunk, is included in Hollis's *Practical Exercise Therapy* (1981).

*Progression*

When axial fixation is used to strengthen weak muscles a natural progression consists of introducing a simple weight-and-pulley circuit to provide the working muscles with graduated resistance. Free exercises of the appropriate grade can be used to supplement this training. They can also be used to provide progression in mobility.

## Supported Exercises

Supported exercises take place in the horizontal plane and are similar to axial suspension movements. The affected part of the body is supported by the buoyancy of water, a highly polished re-education board or ball-bearing skates. The prime mover muscles are indirectly assisted by the counter-balancing of all gravity stresses.

When a polished board is used movement can take place in an oblique plane by tilting the board to the required angle. In this way it is possible to use gravity to give assistance or resistance to the prime movers.

*Progression*

By free exercises of the appropriate grade.

## REFERENCE

Hollis M. (1981) *Practical Exercise Therapy*, 2nd ed. Oxford, Blackwell Scientific Publications.

# 4. Resisted exercises

Resisted exercises are those in which the prime mover muscles work against the resistance of some outside force. Resistance may be provided by (a) Apparatus: weight-and-pulley circuits, weights, springs and elastic substances; (b) Malleable materials; (c) Water; (d) the Therapist; and (e) the Patient.

In applying resistance to muscles four rules must be observed:

1. It must be given smoothly from the beginning to the end of the movement.

2. Whenever possible it should be applied to the moving part so that it exerts pressure on the surface of the skin facing the direction of the movement. In this way the exteroceptors are stimulated and movement is facilitated.

3. It should diminish gradually from the beginning to the end of the movement, so as to conform to the physiological principle that muscles are capable of exerting their greatest force when they are fully extended, and that as they shorten their force diminishes.

4. A brief period of complete relaxation should follow each muscular effort.


## 1. WEIGHT-AND-PULLEY RESISTANCE

Theoretically, weight-and-pulley resistance is capable of being applied to any of the main muscle groups, including those of the trunk. In practice, however, it is usually limited to the muscles of the upper and lower limbs: on average, it is more used for the knee extensors than for any other muscle group.

With a weight-and-pulley circuit the leverage of resistance decreases as the line of application of the force approaches the fulcrum. In other words, the maximum effect of a given resistance on muscles is obtained when it is arranged at right angles to the long axis of the moving limb; the nearer the force is applied in line with the long axis the less is the resistance offered to the muscles.

*Figs.* 17 and 18 indicate the principle of diminishing resistance as applied to the extensor muscles of the knee. *Figs.* 18 and 19 show how relaxation for the working muscles is obtained in the starting and finishing positions by the use

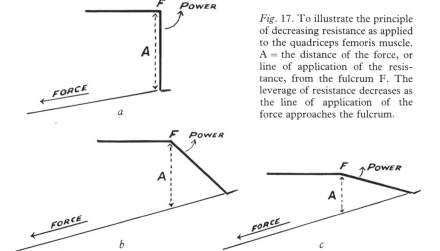

*Fig.* 17. To illustrate the principle of decreasing resistance as applied to the quadriceps femoris muscle. A = the distance of the force, or line of application of the resistance, from the fulcrum F. The leverage of resistance decreases as the line of application of the force approaches the fulcrum.

of a relaxation stop (RS). The stop consists of one of the wooden runners of the lower pulley circuit.

Sometimes a rectangular-shaped piece of wood provided with three holes for the cord is employed as a relaxation stop. *See* inset, *Fig.* 22, p. 25. When used with very heavy weights, however, this type of stop tends to shift along the cord when it strikes the pulley sheave at the end of a movement.

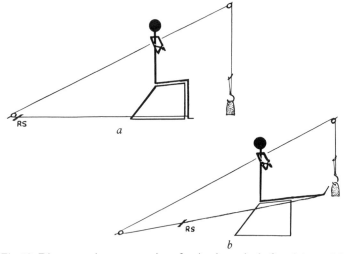

*Fig.* 18. Diagrammatic representation of a simple method of applying weight-and-pulley resistance to the quadriceps femoris muscle. RS represents the relaxation stop which frees the muscle from resistance 'pull' in the resting position.

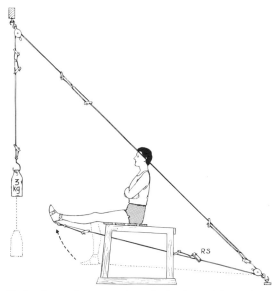

*Fig.* 19. Resisted exercise: extension of the knee joint using a simple triangular-shaped weight-and-pulley circuit. The surface of the fixation bench should slope slightly backwards, as shown; in addition a wooden wedge, covered with felt or foam rubber, is generally used under the thigh. Note the relaxation stop RS.

The triangular-shaped weight-and-pulley circuit for the extensors of the knee needs a high ceiling (at least 4·2 m) for the overhead pulley; otherwise the patient's shoulder obstructs the main connecting cord. An alternative type of circuit which can be used when the ceiling height is limited is shown in *Fig.* 20. It has the disadvantage of needing a third pulley, which increases frictional resistance.

Both circuits can be modified to give specific resistance to the vastus medialis component of the quadriceps femoris muscle, which is active throughout the last 10 to 20 per cent of knee extension. Vastus medialis not only determines knee stability, but is particularly responsible for the inner range of knee movement (Williams and Warwick, 1980).

The modification consists of attaching an additional pulley to the floor in such a position that it lies immediately beneath the ankle when the knee joint is extended, as shown in *Fig.* 21. The altered direction of pull achieved in this way automatically increases the resistance offered to the quadriceps action in full knee extension.

The disadvantage of the modified circuit is that resistance is offered only throughout the last 30° of knee extension, and the important middle range of movement is neglected. To overcome this difficulty a special piece of apparatus (known as the 'Constant-resistance-through-range Apparatus' or

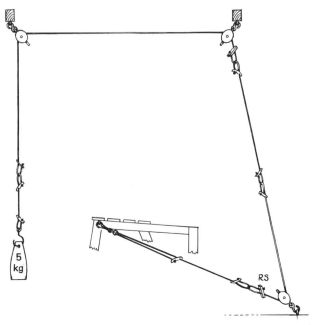

*Fig.* 20. An alternative type of weight-and-pulley circuit for the quadriceps femoris muscle. It is used when ceiling height is limited and the triangular circuit cannot be employed.

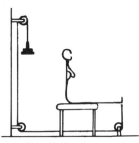

*Fig.* 21. Schematic representation of a simple method of modifying a weight-and-pulley circuit to give specific resistance to the vastus medialis component of the quadriceps femoris muscle.

'CRTRA') has been designed to give constant resistance throughout the entire range of knee flexion and extension with very low friction.

This piece of apparatus formed part of a comparative study of three types of apparatus used for strengthening the quadriceps femoris muscle dynamically (Butler and Kepson, 1980). The apparatus (consisting of a bench which incorporates a lever system linked by a large wooden disc to the weight load) was found to be effective both for exercise and testing purposes. Trials have shown that if the disc were replaced by another shape, for example elliptical, 'the resistance could be increased towards the end of range of quadriceps to work the vastus medialis more, or to increase the resistance at any part of the range as dictated by needs' (Butler and Kepson, 1980).

Weight-and-pulley circuits are an effective means of redeveloping the muscle groups of the elbow and shoulder joints. *Fig.* 22 shows a circuit arranged to give resistance to the abductors of the shoulder. The circuit can also be used to provide resistance for the flexors and extensors of the elbow, and the elevators of the shoulder girdle.

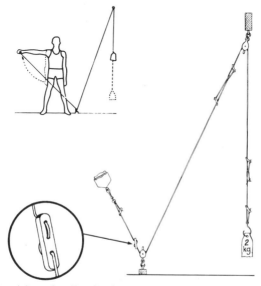

*Fig.* 22. A weight-and-pulley circuit arranged to give resistance to the abductor muscles of the shoulder joint. The circuit can also be used to provide resistance for the muscles of the elbow and the elevators of the shoulder girdle.

Weight-and-pulley resistance can be combined most successfully with axial suspension in providing early strengthening exercises for the main muscle groups of the hip joint, in particular the abductors and extensors. The combined systems can also be used in much the same way with the shoulder muscles.

## Equipment

Weight-and-pulley circuits can be constructed without much difficulty or expense, as indicated by the examples illustrated here. They can be rigged up in the gymnasium or, preferably, in a special pulley room.

In designing or arranging a weight-and-pulley circuit it is important to remember that the patient must not only be able to observe the moving weight throughout the exercise but reach it without difficulty, so that he is capable of adjusting the amount of resistance used and feels fully involved in his treatment programme. Both these factors are of considerable psychological value.

Shaped canvas sandbags with metal eyelets or rings for the weight hook make convenient weights. Bags graded in weight between 125 g and 5 kg are necessary (p. 28). Sometimes metal weights are used instead; they are placed in an open-topped canvas bag equipped with strong metal rings for the weight hook.

Using separate lengths of cord over individual pulley sheaves, as shown in *Figs.* 19 and 22, instead of utilizing one long length of cord for the entire circuit, is economical. When they show signs of fraying and wear, which add to frictional resistance, these short lengths of cord can be replaced quickly by disconnecting the runners.

Specialized pieces of weight-and-pulley equipment which provide a variety of resisted movements for different muscle groups are available from a number of manufacturers of physiotherapy equipment. Most are highly priced.

The 'Quadriceps Bench' manufactured by the Nottingham Medical Equipment Company has been designed to give resistance to the knee extensors through a leverage system rather than by the employment of a weight-and-pulley circuit. The resistance force is applied to the lower leg by means of a padded cross bar which is attached to a swinging arm fitted with removable weights. The cross bar can be positioned along the arm at any point between ankle and knee. This form of adjustment enables the apparatus to be used after injuries where the stability of the lower third of the tibia does not allow a resistance force to be applied to the ankle region, as is usual.

## 2. RESISTANCE BY WEIGHTS

Resistance by weights is a simple and effective method of strengthening muscles. It is capable of being applied to any of the main muscle groups, but in practice (as with weight-and-pulley resistance) is used chiefly for the muscles of the limbs.

The equipment required ranges from metal discs of a known weight, which are employed with weight boots, dumb-bells and barbells, to bags of sand or shot. The weight marked on each bag should represent the combined weight of contents and cover.

Weight resistance has the disadvantage that, when it is applied to the muscle groups of the limbs in the standing and sitting positions, it *increases* from the beginning to the end of all movements made within an arc of 90° from the vertical plane; this is because the perpendicular distance between the line of pull of the weight and the moving joint increases (*Fig.* 23). On the other hand, when weight resistance is applied to the muscles of the limbs in

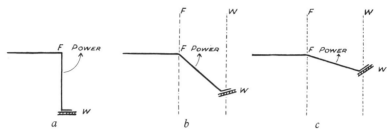

*Fig.* 23. Schematic representation of weight resistance applied to the quadriceps femoris muscle in sitting. The resistance increases from the beginning to the end of the knee extension movement because the perpendicular distance between the line of pull of the weight and the moving joint increases.

the lying position, it *decreases* from the beginning to the end of all movements which are made within an arc of 90° from the horizontal plane, because the perpendicular distance between the line of pull of the weight and the moving joint decreases, e.g. straight leg raising through 50° with a loaded weight boot attached to the foot, and flexion of the shoulder joint through 90° with extended elbow and a dumb-bell held in the hand.

In applying weight resistance to the muscles of the trunk the same factors hold good. Compare *Trunk raising forwards (barbell held at chest level)* from *fixed lying*, and *Trunk lowering forwards (barbell held behind neck)* from *stride-standing*. In the first example the resistance decreases and in the second it increases.

## Equipment

When the muscles of the lower limb are exercised a light alloy weight boot (e.g. Variweight boot) is worn on the foot with a short rod positioned in the slots provided in the sole plate; the metal discs are held securely in place on the rod by two collars with adjustable screws. *Fig.* 24 shows a loaded weight boot in position for the start of resisted knee extension. The weight rod is positioned directly under the ankle.

In calculating the weight to be used for resistance it is essential to know both the weight of the boot and straps, and the rod. The Variweight boot and straps weigh 500 g, and the rod and collars 454 g.

Although metal rods are obtainable as standard equipment it is cheaper to use short lengths of gas piping. These improvised rods provide extremely strong and lightweight forms of support for the weight discs.

The straps and buckles (or Velcro fastenings) securing the weight boot to the foot must be inspected regularly. After considerable use the straps and Velcro grips often fail to hold the boot firmly in place, and must be renewed.

When weights are used to provide resistance for the muscles of the upper limb a loaded weight rod is held in the hand; alternatively, a dumb-bell is used.

Resisted trunk movements necessitate either the use of a barbell or a canvas bag (containing sandbag or metal weights) which is positioned on the chest or back and held in place by long straps.

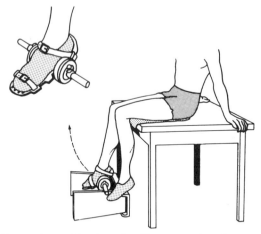

*Fig.* 24. The starting position for resisted knee extension when a weight boot is used. Some form of support should be employed to relieve the knee ligaments of strain in the resting position: here a wall-bar stool has been used for this purpose. Ideally the surface of the fixation bench should have a slight backward slope, and a wedge-shaped pad should be used under the thigh or thighs.

Canvas-covered sandbags are available in different sizes and shapes; they can also be made up fairly easily. In general, the bags need to be capable of being strapped in position without difficulty. The saddle type of bag, which consists of a firm strip of canvas with slots at either end for weights, is particularly useful. When used for leg exercises from lying (e.g. straight leg raising) it is often modified by the addition of a canvas loop attached to the front edge. In positioning the bag the saddle area is placed over the anterior aspect of the ankle and the loop slipped over the foot. This provides a sound anchorage during movement.

Flat, rectangular-shaped PVC-covered sandbags can also be strapped in position without difficulty. In general, the shaped canvas sandbag, with a metal ring or eyelet incorporated into the upper end, is limited to use in activities where it can be suspended easily.

Whatever type of bag is used a fairly wide range of weights is necessary, e.g. 125 g, 250 g, 0·5 kg, 1 kg, 2 kg, 3 kg and 5 kg.

'Portabell' weighted bands are sometimes used in place of weight bags, and have the advantage of being extremely easy to apply. The bands incorporate pockets filled with lead shot, and are held in place round a limb with Velcro fastenings. Two weights of band are available: $1\frac{3}{4}$ lb and $2\frac{1}{2}$ lb.

## STRENGTH PROGRESSION TECHNIQUES

In progressing exercises where weight or weight-and-pulley resistance is used the therapist has to bear in mind the fact that although he is aiming at increasing muscle strength and hypertrophy he is dealing in general with weak and atrophied muscles and traumatized joints. The very heavy weights and comparatively low repetitions used by bodybuilders and weight-lifters in their training programmes, although ideal for boosting the strength of normal muscles, have frequently to be modified considerably or they may well prove harmful. On the other hand, if the weights used are kept to a very low figure, with repetitions at a comparatively high level, there is little chance of achieving muscle hypertrophy; the technique will promote the development of endurance rather than the development of strength.

It is difficult, if not impossible, to give a foolproof technique of progression for all conditions and all phases of recovery. It is possible, however, to describe techniques that have been found valuable over a considerable period of time.

### Early Technique

It is safe to exercise weak muscles against an *initial* resistance of 25 per cent of the greatest weight which they can lift ten times in succession at a normal controlled rate without marked discomfort or fatigue. This ten-times weight is known as the '10 Repetition Maximum' or '10 RM'. The smaller weight is known as the 'Minimum Exercise Weight'.

On the first day of treatment the muscles are exercised against the minimum exercise weight for a period of 4 minutes, a brief rest pause being taken half-way through the session. Thus the patient exercises continuously for 2 minutes, rests until his muscles feel capable of exercising again, and then exercises for another 2 minutes.

*Progression in strength* is achieved very gradually by increasing the minimum exercise weight by 125 or 250 g, when the patient finds that he has grown accustomed to the weight he has been lifting, and the effort no longer tires the muscles to any appreciable extent. Some measure of fatigue is, of course, unavoidable if the weight used is of the degree necessary to achieve muscle hypertrophy.

The weight increase is continued in this way until the resistance employed is found to be approximately 50 per cent of the 10 Repetition Maximum (which will also have increased). The minimum exercise weight is then kept at this level until treatment is discontinued, the actual weight used being increased in direct proportion to the 10 RM. This weight must be checked twice weekly to ascertain if it may be increased.

*Progression in time* is brought about by increasing the exercise time by 1 minute each day until the patient is exercising with the minimum exercise weight for 15 minutes before the rest pause, and 15 minutes after it. The length of the rest pause naturally depends on the degree of muscle fatigue.

On occasions it is extremely helpful if two exercise periods are organized daily, provided that they are adequately spaced to avoid undue fatigue. A morning and afternoon session is ideal, although often difficult to achieve.

It is important that the patient should be encouraged to participate fully in his training programme. Whenever possible (and this will obviously depend on his intelligence and attitude towards recovery) he should not only be responsible for increasing resistance levels, but keep his own check on the weights used and the number of minutes for which he exercises each day. All this prevents the exercise régime from becoming tedious and automatic.

A realistic way of persuading patients to maintain records of their own progress is to install a wall-mounted blackboard in the gymnasium or pulley room for this purpose.

### More Advanced Technique

When the muscles have reached a satisfactory state of redevelopment a more advanced exercise technique, which combines both power and endurance training, may be used; it can also be used in cases where a more strenuous initial exercise programme can be tolerated. This form of training has the advantage of preparing the muscles for normal working conditions: short periods of activity against maximum stresses and prolonged periods of work against minimum stresses.

The technique is much the same as that previously described, with the exception that two sets of lifts with the 10 RM are incorporated into the training schedule. Thus—

> 10 lifts with 10 RM
> Training period with minimum
>     exercise weight, with half-time
>     rest pause.
> 10 lifts with 10 RM

It is important to note that although the patient may not be able to perform the full number of repetitions during the second set of lifts with the 10 RM he must be prepared to attempt as many lifts as possible. Unless this is done maximum hypertrophy will not result. Expert supervision and care are most important in this type of training. An enthusiastic patient may attempt too much and bring about muscular strain or joint effusion.

### EXERCISE TECHNIQUE

All movements must be performed in a smooth controlled manner so that the muscles work concentrically, statically and then excentrically. Thus, in strengthening the quadriceps femoris muscle from a sitting position on a fixation bench, the patient extends the knee to its full extent, 'holds' it in this position for a moment, and then allows it to return to the starting position. After a momentary pause the movement is repeated. (*See Figs.* 19 and 24, pp. 23 and 28.)

In exercising the muscles of the limbs it is usual to limit resistance to the affected limb only. When the limbs are equal in strength, however, the sound limb may be exercised against resistance also. In practice this is seldom necessary, because the sound limb will be exercised adequately when other aspects of the patient's rehabilitation programme are carried out—during sessions devoted to specific and general exercises and in recreational activities.

## ASSESSING MUSCLE STRENGTH

In redeveloping weak muscles it is important to test periodically the 10 repetition maximum weight of the corresponding sound muscle group, so that the relative weakness of the affected muscle group may be ascertained, and a standard set for the patient to aim at. The result is expressed as a fraction: Left/Right = 9 kg/4 kg, in the case of a weak right quadriceps femoris muscle. In dealing with the trunk muscles, where this type of comparison is not possible, a known standard is determined by testing out a number of normal subjects.

The 10 RM weight of the affected and corresponding sound muscle groups should be recorded twice weekly and plotted as a graph. These tests not only form a reliable guide to progress but are extremely instructive. In addition, the incontrovertible evidence that muscles are becoming stronger is a great encouragement to both patient and therapist, especially in cases where progress is slow.

Each time the tests are made the same weight apparatus or weight-and-pulley circuit should be used. This is particularly important when using pulley circuits, because the frictional resistance offered by individual pulley sheaves varies considerably. The same precautions apply when weights and weight-and-pulley circuits are used for exercise purposes.

## MAKING A TEST

In assessing the 10 RM of a muscle group it is important for the patient to avoid trying out too many different poundages before arriving at the correct one. The muscles will become so fatigued by this preliminary work that it will be almost impossible to make an accurate test.

A useful method of determining the weight is for the therapist to select a weight which he considers to be a reasonable resistance for the purposes of the test, and then ask the patient to make a small movement against its resistance. In this way the patient can try the effect of the weight on his muscles without using them sufficiently to produce fatigue. If he finds the weight is too much, or too little (bearing in mind a series of ten repetitions), the poundage is adjusted accordingly and the test repeated.

When the patient thinks that the correct weight has been found, he tries the ten full movements against it. If the patient and the therapist are satisfied after this that the weight is the right one, no further tests are made. If they are not satisfied with the result, the muscles are allowed to rest until they are ready for exercise again and a further test is made.

For assessment purposes a test with a One Repetition Maximum (the greatest weight which can be lifted once only by the muscle group) is sometimes used when muscle development has reached a satisfactory level and there is no danger of irritating a traumatized joint.

*Myometer*

Recently a hand-held myometer (*Fig.* 25), which monitors muscle strength, has been developed for clinical use.★ Basically, the instrument is a device to measure the peak force applied by the examiner in resisting, and overcoming, the maximum contraction of a muscle group. The force is expressed in kilograms and the instrument has a recording range of 0·1–30·0 kg, which may be seen on the digital readout display.

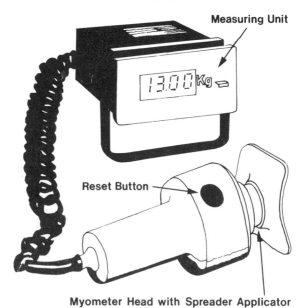

**Measuring Unit**

**Reset Button**

**Myometer Head with Spreader Applicator**

*Fig.* 25. A hand-held myometer for monitoring muscle strength.

★ Penny and Giles Transducers Ltd., Christchurch, Dorset.

The myometer head, which carries a spreader applicator, utilizes the measuring element of a standard Penny and Giles transducer. The method of measuring consists of the deflection of a diaphragm in air; the deflection moves the wiper of a conductive plastic potentiometer with a life expectancy of 100 000 000 operations.

To some degree the range of usefulness of the instrument is limited by the strength of the examiner in resisting the contractions of the patient's muscles. He needs to assume an extremely stable position when using the myometer, especially when testing large muscle groups such as the hamstrings and quadriceps femoris.

Methods of measuring muscle strength and fatigue, including the use of myometer and strain gauge, were described by Edwards and Hyde (1977). The evaluation of voluntary-muscle function by means of a hand-held dynamometer was also the subject of a paper by Edwards and McDonnell (1974).

*Fixed Myometer*

A simple myometer designed specifically to test the strength of the quadriceps femoris muscle during the final degrees of knee extension has been designed by Mr J. V. Gough, Director of Rehabilitation, Pinderfields General Hospital.

The myometer has the advantage of being firmly stabilized during testing by a rigid frame which is positioned over the patient's lower leg. A padded movable applicator, which makes contact with the upper third of the tibia, is linked to the measuring device. This consists of a simple, oil-filled bellows and a pressure gauge. Compression of the bellows during extension of the knee operates the gauge.

## OTHER METHODS OF RESISTANCE TRAINING

The resistance training methods described in the previous section are based on those originally formulated by Nicoll and Colson over the period 1940–43 as part of a pioneer scheme of medical rehabilitation for injured miners in the UK (Nicoll, 1941, 1943).

Later, other methods of resistance training (based on the heavy resistance techniques used by bodybuilders and weight-lifters) were developed from time to time. Three main systems, known by the names of their originators, are in use today: DeLorme and Watkins technique (1951); Zinovieff or Oxford technique (1951); and McQueen technique (1954).

### Heavy Resistance Systems

The heavy resistance systems are mainly intended for use with weights, although they may be used equally well with weight-and-pulley circuits.

Common to the three techniques is the 10 Repetition Maximum (10 RM), the maximum weight which can be lifted by the weak muscle group for ten repetitions only. For example, in assessing the 10 RM of a weak quadriceps femoris muscle, the patient assumes a sound starting position on a fixation bench, with a weight boot strapped to his foot, and observes the following schedule. Starting with the weight of the boot and its loading bar, and increasing by small amounts (e.g. 0·5–2·5 kg), he lifts each weight ten times at a normal controlled rate. The weight which requires the maximum muscular effort to perform the ten repetition series of lifts is taken as the 10 RM.

### DeLorme and Watkins 'Fractional' Technique

The 10 RM resistance is increased *gradually* over 3 sets of repetitions. Thus—

> 1st set: 10 lifts with half 10 RM
> 2nd set: 10 lifts with three-quarters 10 RM
> 3rd set: 10 lifts with 10 RM

Thirty lifts are carried out daily, four times a week. Each week the 10 RM is progressed.

COMMENT

The system has the advantage of being extremely straightforward and simple to follow. Considerable care is needed in assessing the initial 10 RM or the patient may be disheartened by finding it almost impossible to achieve the final full set of lifts.

### Zinovieff (Oxford) Technique

The 10 RM resistance is *decreased* gradually over ten sets of repetitions. Thus—

> 1st set: 10 lifts with 10 RM
> 2nd set: 10 lifts with 10 RM *subtracting* 0·5 kg
> 3rd set: 10 lifts with 10 RM *subtracting* 1 kg
> 4th set: 10 lifts with 10 RM *subtracting* 1·5 kg
> 5th set: 10 lifts with 10 RM *subtracting* 2 kg
> 6th set: 10 lifts with 10 RM *subtracting* 2·5 kg
> 7th set: 10 lifts with 10 RM *subtracting* 3 kg
> 8th set: 10 lifts with 10 RM *subtracting* 3·5 kg
> 9th set: 10 lifts with 10 RM *subtracting* 4 kg
> 10th set: 10 lifts with 10 RM *subtracting* 4·5 kg

A hundred lifts are carried out daily, five times weekly. At each exercise session an attempt is made to progress the 10 RM.

COMMENT

Because of the number of individual sets of repetitions which must be followed (all with different weights) many patients and their therapists find the system irritating. The constant changing of weights is also extremely time-consuming.

## McQueen Technique

The 10 RM resistance is *maintained*, without addition or subtraction, over four sets of lifts. Thus—

> 1st set: 10 lifts with 10 RM
> 2nd set: 10 lifts with 10 RM
> 3rd set: 10 lifts with 10 RM
> 4th set: 10 lifts with 10 RM

Forty lifts are carried out three times a week. Progression is achieved by attempting to increase the 10 RM every one to two weeks.

COMMENT

The system is straightforward but the overall work load is heavy; the patient needs considerable determination to follow it satisfactorily. As with the DeLorme and Watkins technique care is needed in assessing the initial 10 RM, or overloading of the muscles may result and the patient will experience difficulty in completing the final set of lifts.

## Other Heavy Resistance Systems

A number of other heavy resistance systems have been developed by therapists and physical educationists with specialized experience of weight training. In these systems the RM varies between 1 and 10, with a 6 or 8 RM being common. The number of repetitions and sets of lifts varies also, e.g. 6, 8 or 10. For maximum muscle development six repetitions, in six sets of lifts, is advocated (total of 36 lifts).

Many experts in the field of weight training consider that the widely accepted figure of 10 lifts per set could well be replaced by a lower number, and suggest 6 as a useful compromise. They emphasize that the patient's concentration and maximum effort wanes over long lifting sessions.

## Limitation of Heavy Resistance Systems

Heavy resistance techniques need to be used with considerable care in exercise therapy. In general, they are more applicable to the intermediate and late phases of recovery after injury and disease than to any other stage. If used in the earlier phases considerable modification is frequently necessary to avoid muscle strain and joint reaction.

## 3. RESISTANCE BY SPRINGS

Springs, rubber elastic strands and various compressible materials, such as Dunlopillo and Sorbo rubber, all possess the property of elasticity and are used to provide different forms of therapeutic resistance.

### Long Spiral Springs

Long spiral (or long tension) springs, being readily extensible, offer resistance to the working muscle group as they are stretched, and assistance to the return movement as they recoil. Alternatively, the recoil movement may be controlled by excentric action of the working muscles (*Fig.* 26).

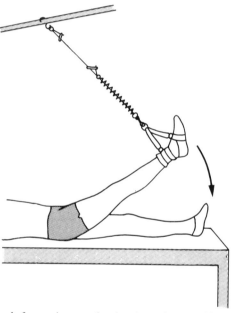

*Fig.* 26. Method of arranging a cord and spring unit to provide resistance for the extensor muscles of the hip in lying. The angle of pull is critical. So also is the weight resistance of the spring used; it must be capable of supporting the lower limb in addition to providing resistance for the hip extensors.

Resistance given by these springs can be extremely useful, but it has two disadvantages. It is not physiologically sound: resistance from springs is always weakest at the beginning of the movement, when the muscles are extended, and strongest at the end of the movement when the muscles are shortened; and it cannot be accurately assessed.

. The weight resistance of a tension spring depends on the type of material and thickness of wire from which it is constructed and the average diameter of the coils.

In general, standard spiral springs are still (1982) graded in pounds. They are available in four main weights: 10 lb (4·5 kg), 20 lb (9 kg), 30 lb (13·6 kg) and 40 lb (18·1 kg). The weight marked on each spring represents the weight resistance or poundage offered when it is stretched to its full length. A safety tape inside the spring becomes taut when the predetermined point is reached and checks overstretching and damage to the coils.

When a specific weight of spring is not available two springs (each of half the weight required) can be used in parallel combination to provide the required resistance (*Fig.* 27a). For example, two 30 lb (13·6 kg) springs arranged in parallel are equal to a 60 lb (27·2 kg) spring.

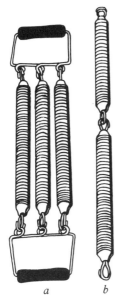

*Fig.* 27. Springs arranged in parallel and springs linked in series.

*a*        *b*

Conversely, arranging two springs of equal 'weight' end-to-end, or in series (*Fig.* 27b), can be used to produce a spring of half the weight resistance, provided the springs are extended through the range required to extend *one* to its full limit. In practice, the double length of spring produced by this method of linkage can be cumbersome.

## Arranging Spring Resistance

In arranging spring resistance a number of points must be observed:

1. A stable and comfortable starting position must be used which enables the resisted movements to be isolated correctly.

2. The spring must be of the correct weight resistance for the muscles; in some exercises it must also be capable of supporting the weight of the moving part (*see Fig.* 26).

3. The positioning of the spring in relation to the moving part requires considerable care. The arrangement used must not only ensure that the spring is slightly stretched at the start of the movement, but offers effective resistance throughout the required range of movement.

4. The connecting links that attach the spring to the fixed point and the moving part must be sufficiently strong to withstand considerable stresses. For many movements, particularly those of a wide range nature, it is necessary to increase the distance between the fixed point and the spring; the link then consists of a suspension cord with a single runner for adjustment purposes.

The link between the spring and the moving part consists of a spring-loaded hook with swivel and some form of sling; the self-locking 3-ring sling shown in *Fig.* 26 is widely used. (*See also Fig.* 16, p. 19.) For some arm movements a handle attached to the spring is used in place of a sling.

## Other Types of Springs

*Short Tension Springs*

Short tension springs of a high resistance level offer minimum extensibility, and are not used in resistance training. They are sometimes employed in suspension therapy to provide buoyancy when a heavy part of the body, such as the pelvis or trunk, has to be supported in sling suspension for a fairly long period of time. The springs are then arranged to form a link between the overhead support and the suspension cords.

*Small Compressible Springs*

These springs form the resistance element in the familiar hand grip unit which is used to improve the coarse gripping action of the hand. Another similar device for improving grip consists of a Z-shaped spring made from flat steel.

## Elastic Strands and Sorbo Rubber

Rubber elastic strands of various widths are sometimes used in place of long spiral springs; they are especially useful for providing light resistance. Rubber elastic has the disadvantage of not being particularly durable.

Sorbo rubber, being both compressible and extensible, is extremely useful in providing light resistance for improving the gripping action of the hand. Rubber balls and sponges of different shapes and sizes provide useful variations.

## Progression of Spring Resistance

With spring resistance an accurate and precise progression in strength is not possible. A very approximate degree of progression is achieved by increasing the 'weight' of the spring or springs employed, e.g. by replacing a 10 lb (4·5 kg) spring by a 20 lb (9 kg) spring, or increasing the number of springs arranged in parallel.

## 4. RESISTANCE BY MALLEABLE MATERIALS

Moulding putty, clay, Plasticine or wet sand into various simple shapes provides both resistance for the hand muscles and some degree of mobilizing activity for the joints.

This type of resistance is limited and often employed as an introductory to the more realistic functional activities provided by an occupational therapy workshop, e.g. stool seating, which provides both narrow and wide grips, printing and woodwork (padded handles being used for some of the equipment, such as planes and sanding blocks), model making and wrought iron work.

Remedial games which encourage grip complement these workshop activities. Competitive blow football (necessitating the squeezing of the rubber bulb of a syringe to blow out air to propel a ping-pong ball along a table) is extremely useful and popular. So also is bar football: the handles used to activate the 'players' can be adapted to offer various types of grip. These games are described and illustrated in Wynn Parry's *Rehabilitation of the Hand,* 3rd ed.

## 5. RESISTANCE BY WATER

The degree of resistance offered by water depends on the surface area of the part moved and the rate of movement. Increasing the surface area automatically necessitates the displacement of a larger volume of water and leads to an increase in resistance. Similarly, an increase in the speed of movement produces an associated increase of resistance. This is largely due to the turbulence associated with a more rapid movement, positive pressure being created in the direction of the movement and a negative, or drag force, behind it.

In pool therapy, when the body is floating horizontally in the water with buoyancy providing support, it is comparatively easy to enlarge the surface area of a limb by the use of a small float, such as a swim ring or cork or polystyrene block. When the arm is exercised a simple progression can be achieved by the patient using the flat of his hand (rather than the edge) as he moves the limb through the water. A more advanced progression consists of his holding a paddle or bat, or similar flat object, in the hand during movement. This not only increases the length of the lever but adds effectively to the surface area of the arm.

When movements are made in a *downward* direction from a floating horizontal position the upthrust of buoyancy provides resistance. 'The maximum upthrust is experienced when the limb is at right angles to the buoyant force. The effect is reduced the nearer the moving part gets to the vertical. If the range of movement goes beyond 90°, buoyancy will no longer be providing resistance and the movement beyond the vertical becomes buoyancy assisted. Flexion of the hip is an example (*Fig.* 28*a*). The starting position is prone lying at the edge of a stretcher or over the exercise bars so that the hip is free. The patient brings the leg downwards and forwards into flexion. Only the first part of the movement (outer-to-middle range for the hip flexors) is resisted by buoyancy. The rest of the movement (middle-to-inner range) is assisted.

'Similarly, when doing knee extension, the full effect of the resistance will be felt when the lower leg is horizontal, at right angles to the buoyant force (inner range for the quadriceps) (*Fig.* 28*b*).

'The muscle work can be increased in the usual ways, by increasing speed, duration, length of lever and resistance. Extra resistance can be provided by

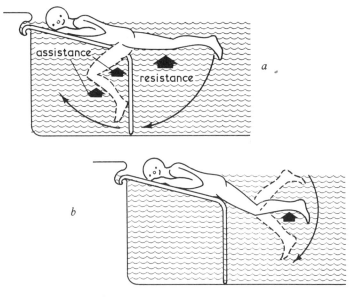

*Fig.* 28. *a*, Upthrust of buoyancy used as a resistance for the hip flexors from a prone lying position at the edge of a stretcher or over the exercise bars. Only the first part of the movement (outer to middle range for hip flexors) is resisted by buoyancy. The rest of the movement is assisted. *b*, Buoyancy used as resistance for the knee extensors: same starting position as described in *Fig.* 28*a*. The full effect of the resistance is felt when the lower leg is horizontal, at right angles to the buoyant force (inner range for quadriceps). (Illustrations reproduced from 'Basic hydrotherapy', *Physiotherapy* (1981), **67**, 258–262, by kind permission of the author and the Editor of the Journal.)

using floats which the patient has to push down into the water. These floats alter the shape and density of the moving part. Very powerful strengthening exercises can be devised in this way, but instability is the problem, and the therapist may well be working as hard as the patient, to hold him down.'*

It should be noted that during *upward* return movements to the horizontal buoyancy minimizes or cancels out much of the resistance.

## 6. MANUAL RESISTANCE

Resistance by the therapist is useful in cases where the muscles are extremely weak or where suitable resistance apparatus is not available. Smooth controlled pressure should be applied by the hand throughout the movement and, whenever possible, the therapist's stance should be in the line of the movement. This is especially important when moderate or strong resistance is given; the body weight and the thrusting action of the legs can then be used to advantage.

Manual resistance of this type has the disadvantage that it cannot be assessed accurately. It is also not possible for the therapist to give or maintain the amount of resistance necessary to strengthen muscles to the degree required for heavy occupations.

In *self-resistance* the patient resists his own movements with a sound limb. For example, in high sitting, with the ankles crossed, the extensors of one knee can be resisted by the weight and pressure of the other leg. Similarly, various movements of the wrist, elbow and shoulder of one limb can be resisted successfully by the hand of the opposite limb.

Self-resistance is obviously extremely limited. Accurate assessment of strength is not possible and only a relatively few muscle groups can be treated.

## REFERENCES

Butler P. and Kepson G. (1980) Quadriceps strengthening: a comparative study of three types of apparatus for strengthening the quadriceps femoris muscle dynamically. *Physiotherapy* **66**, 82–85.

DeLorme T. L. (1945) Restoration of muscle power by heavy resistance exercises. *J. Bone Joint Surg.* **27**, 646–667.

DeLorme T. L. and Watkins A. L. (1945) Technics of progressive resistance exercises. *Arch. Phys. Med.* **29**, 263–273.

DeLorme T. L. and Watkins A. L. (1951) *Progressive Resistance Exercises: Technique and Medical Application.* New York, Appleton-Century-Crofts.

Dick F. W. (1968) A review of recent studies pertaining to strength. *Br. J. Sports Med.* **4**, 35–41.

* This description and the accompanying illustrations are taken from 'Basic hydrotherapy' (*Physiotherapy*, Sept., 1981) by Anne Golland, MCSP.

Edwards R. H. T. and Hyde S. (1977) Method of measuring muscle strength and fatigue. *Physiotherapy*, **63**, 51–55.

Edwards R. H. T. and McDonnell M. (1974) Handheld dynamometer for evaluating voluntary muscle function. *Lancet* **2**, 757.

Nicoll E. A. (1941) Rehabilitation of the injured. *Br. Med. J.* **1**, 501–506.

Nicoll E. A. (1943) Principles of exercise therapy. *Br. Med. J.* **1**, 747–750.

McQueen I. (1954) Recent advances in the technique of progressive resistance exercises. *Br. Med. J.* **2**, 1193–1198.

Websters B. M. (1982) Factors influencing strength testing and exercise prescription. *Physiotherapy* **68**, 42–44.

Williams P. L. and Warwick R. (1980) *Gray's Anatomy*, 36th ed. Edinburgh, Churchill Livingstone.

Wynn Parry C. B. (1973) *Rehabilitation of the Hand*, 3rd ed. London, Butterworths.

Zinovieff A. (1951) Heavy resistance exercises: the Oxford technique. *Br. J. Phys. Med. Ind. Hyg.* **14**, 129.

# PART 2

# FUNCTIONAL MOVEMENTS

This section describes a number of basic functional movements which are used in the early stages of mobilization and re-education. They are concerned with positioning and moving in bed and on the floor. They also include manœuvres designed to enable patients to move safely through various positions and directions. For example, from lying to sitting, from sitting to standing, and from standing to floor level.

# 5. Movements on the bed or floor

## MOVING ON THE BED FROM SUPINE LYING

### Moving Towards the Head of the Bed  ⬅

The manœuvre is usually carried out from crook lying. The patient raises the pelvis off the supporting surface to the low Bridge position by extension of the hips and spine combined with down-pressure from the arms and shoulder girdle. The body is then moved horizontally towards the head of the bed by a strong thrusting movement from the soles of the feet. This action is often associated with extension of the neck.

In clinical practice, when it is not possible to use both legs, the manœuvre is modified by changing the starting position. The patient flexes the hip and knee of the sound leg until the knee is bent to about 90° with the sole of the foot resting flat on the bed; at the same time he flexes the elbows to a right angle (*Fig. 29a*). He then raises the pelvis off the supporting surface to the low Bridge position by a strong movement of extension of the flexed hip and spine combined with down-pressure from the arms and shoulder girdle (*Fig. 29b*). Strong pressure on the sole of the foot of the bent leg then helps to propel the body horizontally towards the bed head, as previously described.

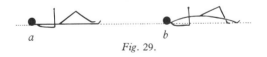

*a*              *b*

*Fig.* 29.

### Moving Down the Bed  ➡

The patient assumes the crook lying position with the elbows flexed to about 90° (*Fig. 30a*). As a preliminary movement he arches the spine strongly with the pelvis remaining on the bed. He then presses down firmly with elbows and head and raises the pelvis slightly clear of the supporting surface (*Fig. 30b*).

He eases the pelvis downwards towards the heels in a relatively small range movement. The active muscles are then relaxed smoothly and the pelvis lowered on to the bed. This sequence of movements is repeated.

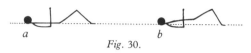

*a*                          *b*

*Fig. 30.*

In practice, if it is not possible for the patient to flex both legs in the starting position, the manœuvre can be carried out successfully using one leg only.

## Moving Across the Bed

The patient takes up the crook lying position with the arms slightly away from the sides and the palms of the hands resting on the bed. He raises the pelvis off the supporting surface (low Bridge position: *Fig. 30b*) and eases it sideways in the required direction. He then lowers the pelvis on to the bed, allows the legs to straighten out, and adjusts the alignment of the upper trunk and head.

It is possible to carry out this manœuvre with one leg in a crook position. When moving to the side of the straight leg it is advisable to place this limb into an *abducted* position, so as to avoid adduction stresses at the hip during the sideways movement. This is particularly important in the postoperative care of a total hip replacement.

## Rolling on to the Left Side

The patient flexes the hip and knee of the right leg until the knee is bent to about 90°, with the sole of the foot resting flat on the bed; the left leg is straight and the left hand grasps the side of the bed with the arm slightly abducted. A simultaneous movement of strong head turning to the left, right arm stretching across the chest—with a firm thrust from the right foot—helps to rotate the whole of the trunk and pelvis to the left.

In this position the flexed right leg lies over the straight left leg. To stabilize the body the left leg is then flexed to the same degree as the right. The patient is then in a modified crook side lying position.

In this posture considerable pressure is exerted on the left shoulder, and some patients, particularly the elderly, may experience considerable discomfort. To avoid this the right hand can be used to press down on the bed and help to manœuvre the arm and shoulder into a comfortable position.

## Assuming Bridge Position

The patient flexes the knees to 90° with the soles of the feet resting on the bed; the legs are slightly astride with the inner borders of the feet about a foot-breadth apart. The arms are slightly away from the sides with the palms of the hands facing downwards. This arrangement of legs and arms ensures a stable starting position (*Fig.* 31*a*).

The pelvis is then raised clear of the supporting surface by strong extension of the hips and thoracolumbar spine with associated knee extension: Bridge position (*Fig.* 31*b*).

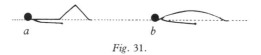

*a*                                    *b*

*Fig.* 31.

The position is widely used for various nursing procedures, e.g. giving of bed-pan and attention to pressure areas. In a modified form (low Bridge) it is widely used as a preliminary to a number of functional movements, as previously described.

In certain clinical conditions when it is not possible to utilize both legs in the crook position the bridging manœuvre can be achieved with one leg crooked. The starting position is then somewhat unstable. To counteract this during movement manual support can be provided under the lumbar spine or buttocks. Another method of providing stability is to support the straight leg with a firm pillow.

### Rolling from Supine to Prone Lying

To roll to the left from supine lying the patient crosses the right ankle over the left; he then brings the left arm close to the left side so that the palm makes contact with the outer side of the thigh. The right shoulder is abducted to 90° with the elbow extended and the palm facing upward. The arm is then swung vigorously across the chest to the left. Simultaneously, the head is turned strongly to the left and the trunk follows the movement.

At the end of this manœuvre the patient lies prone with the left arm under the left thigh and the right arm, with elbow flexed, under the chest. The patient then arches the spine slightly and brings the arms into a comfortable position.

If the patient finds it difficult to achieve prone lying in one main movement, as indicated here, a series of small range rocking movements towards the left can be made with the arm and trunk. They culminate in one definite movement which carries the patient over into prone lying.

Another method of rolling over to the left consists of the patient grasping the left head post of the bed with the right hand, and assisting the trunk movements with a strong pulling action.

In the initial stages of rolling, manual assistance is often helpful. The therapist stands at the side of the bed to which the movement is made.

*N.B.* It is important to note that at the start of the rolling procedure the patient must be positioned so that when he assumes the prone position his body is fully supported by the bed and there is no likelihood of his falling over the edge.


## MANŒUVRES ON THE FLOOR OR BED

### Seat Lifting (to relieve the buttocks of body pressure)

The patient assumes the long sitting position with the trunk inclined slightly backwards and the palms of the hands resting on the supporting surface with the fingers pointing outwards. He then lowers the trunk backwards a few degrees and raises the seat clear of the floor or bed by strong extension of the hips, the hands and heels carrying the total body weight (*Fig.* 32). The seat is then returned to its original position by a reversal of the previous movements.

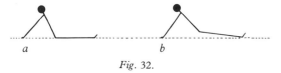

*a*                              *b*

*Fig.* 32.

Seat lifting can also be carried out from the standard long sitting position with the trunk vertical and the arms by the sides. In this case it is easier if the hands are clenched and the weight is taken chiefly on the proximal phalanges.

When seat lifting is carried out on a bed or soft mat (where the supporting surface will yield to hand pressure) it is advisable to use a pair of hand grips mounted on rectangular wooden bases (*Fig.* 33).

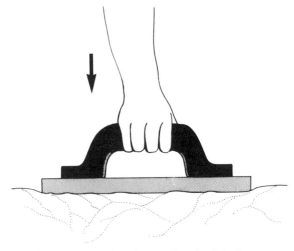

*Fig.* 33. Seat lifting is facilitated by the use of a pair of platform mounted hand grips.

*N.B.* Seat lifting is widely used by patients who have to spend long periods of time in wheelchairs and armchairs to relieve the buttocks of constant pressure. The lifting is done intermittently, the hands grasping the chair arms to accomplish the movement.

### 'Travelling': a simple method of moving the body over a supporting surface

*'Travelling' Forwards* →  →

The patient assumes a modified crook sitting position with the feet about a foot-breadth apart, the trunk inclined backwards and the palms of the hands resting flat on the supporting surface with the fingers pointing outwards (*Fig.* 34a). He then lifts the seat clear of the bed or floor by extending the hips, simultaneously carrying it forwards towards the heels by flexion of the hips and knees (*Fig.* 34b). He then lowers the seat to the supporting surface. (In this position the seat is situated some distance in front of the hands, the knees are well flexed, and the trunk is inclined further back.) (*Fig.* 34c.)

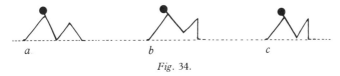

*Fig.* 34.

To progress along the floor or bed the patient places each foot forwards a short distance. He then moves the trunk and arms in the same direction, so that the original starting position is assumed. To cover a wider distance the series of movements is repeated.

*'Travelling' Backwards* ←  ←

This is achieved in much the same fashion as 'travelling' forwards. The movement starts by the patient moving the arms, and then the trunk, in a backward direction. He then lifts the seat off the supporting surface and moves it back towards the arms. Next, he lowers the seat on to the floor or bed. Finally, the feet are moved backwards in turn, so that the original starting position is assumed.

*'Travelling' Sideways*

The patient assumes a modified long sitting position with the feet together, the trunk inclined backwards with the arms away from the sides; the palms of the hands rest on the supporting surface with the fingers pointing outwards.

To move, for example, to the left, the patient leans back slightly and raises the seat clear of the floor or bed, so that the body weight rests entirely on the heels and hands. Simultaneously, he moves the pelvis over to the left. He then lowers the seat to the supporting surface, and moves first the hands with the trunk, and then each foot separately, to the left.

To cover a wider distance this series of movements is repeated.

*N.B.* To avoid pressure on the heels 'travelling' sideways can be carried out from a modified crook sitting position. *See* 'Travelling' forwards.


## MOVEMENTS AT FLOOR LEVEL

### Moving from Sitting on Floor to Sitting on Low Stool

The patient assumes a long sitting position (p. 267) with the spine in contact with the front edge of a stool, 20–25 cm high, positioned behind him. He moves the arms backwards and places the palms of the hands on either side of the stool top, close to the front edge, so that the elbows are well flexed and the shoulder joints fully extended. *Fig.* 35a–b.

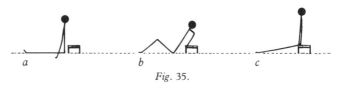

*a*          *b*          *c*

*Fig.* 35.

He then parts the legs slightly and flexes the hips and knees as far as possible with the soles of the feet resting on the floor, each leg being moved in turn. Then, with a strong movement of extension of the arms, reinforced by extension of knees and hips, he lifts the body upwards and backwards so as to bring the buttocks on to the front edge of the stool (low grasp inclined long sitting position) (*Fig.* 35c). From this position he flexes each knee in turn to about 90°, inclines the trunk slightly forwards, and eases the seat back on the stool to a better sitting position (by extension of knees and downward pressure through the straight arms). The hands, in turn, are then moved backwards to a more comfortable position on the stool.


### Assuming Standing from Prone Kneeling with Use of Chair

From prone kneeling (p. 268) with a chair positioned so that the front edge of the seat is close to the head (*Fig.* 36a), the patient first places the palm of each hand on the chair seat. He extends the elbows fully so that the trunk is raised backwards to an oblique position. He then moves one leg forward so that the hip and knee are well flexed and the sole of the foot rests on the floor (*Fig.* 36b).

The body is then raised upwards by a strong thrusting movement of both legs and arms, the toes of the rear foot being dorsiflexed to give added thrust to the movement. In the position reached in this way the arms are vertically over the chair seat, with the trunk more or less horizontal, and the forward leg fully extended. The rear leg, slightly flexed at the knee, rests on the toes (*Fig. 36c*).

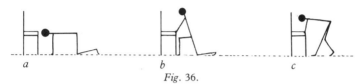

a          b          c

*Fig. 36.*

The rear leg is now carried forwards and placed alongside the other one. The trunk is then raised to the vertical.


## MOVEMENTS IN PRONE LYING ON BED OR MAT

Although many individuals, particularly the elderly and those with limited mobility, find prone lying an uncomfortable position to maintain for any length of time, it is undoubtedly extremely useful in clinical practice. It forms a stable starting position, for example, for encouraging knee flexion following trauma. Similarly, it allows ankle and foot movements to be performed freely with the lower legs maintained in the vertical. This is particularly useful in reducing oedema.

In addition, prone lying not only allows a range of spinal arching movements to be carried out, but forms a natural introductory step to assuming prone kneeling. From prone lying the body can also be manœuvred forwards in a series of 'wriggling' movements.


### Arching

Arching movements of the spine can be facilitated by placing the arms in forearm support position (arms to sides, elbows fully flexed and palms facing downward at shoulder level). The movements are associated with a small degree of elbow extension, the forearms and palms providing a firm base for the movements (*Fig. 37a*).

A wider range of spinal arching, combined with hip extension, can be achieved by placing the palms of the hands by the sides of the trunk at mid-chest level. The elbows are then extended fully during the trunk arching (*Fig. 37b*).

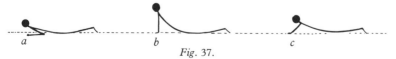

a          b          c

*Fig. 37.*

The palms may also be moved forwards until they are in line with the head. Full elbow extension is then associated only with spinal extension (*Fig.* 37*c*).

Arching is useful in the treatment of postural kyphosis and round shoulders. It is also valuable in the early mobilization of young adults who have spent considerable periods of time in bed following various orthopædic procedures, e.g. fractured shaft of femur treated conservatively with Thomas's splint and traction.


## Assuming Prone Kneeling

With the arms in forearm support position (*see* Arching) the trunk is moved backwards mainly by strong pressure from the arms (full elbow extension with shoulder flexion) combined with flexion of the hips and knees. To bring the arms into the vertical position the hands are 'walked' backwards to the required degree (*Fig.* 38*a–c*).

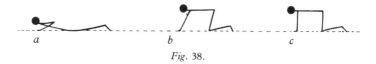

*a*                          *b*                        *c*

*Fig.* 38.


## Leopard Crawl ('Creeping')

This is a somewhat complex and strenuous method of propelling the body in a forward direction along the bed or mat, using a contralateral pattern of movement. It is carried out from a modified forearm support position with the upper arms vertical and the forearms resting on the supporting surface; the hands may be clenched, which is preferable, or the palms may face downward.

The movement starts by the right arm being moved forwards a short distance while the head and trunk are turned to the left. At the same time the left knee is drawn up through 90°, with the inner aspect making contact with the supporting surface. The body is then propelled forwards by a strong levering movement of the right arm (which acts as a prop for the trunk) combined with a thrusting movement from the flexed left leg. To continue the forward progression the same pattern of movement is repeated with the other arm and leg.

This method of progression in prone lying is often beyond the physical capabilities of many elderly and disabled individuals. A similar but less strenuous method of progession consists of a 'wriggling' type of manœuvre.


## 'Wriggling'

This consists of propelling the body in a forward direction along the bed or mat. The patient moves in a wriggling motion with the arms in forearm support position (*see* Arching) and the ankles fully dorsiflexed, so that the plantar surfaces of the toes rest on the supporting surface. The main propulsive action is achieved by alternate hip updrawing (with strong pressure from the toes), followed by alternate elevation of the shoulder girdle.

# 6. Moving from sitting and standing

## MOVING FROM SITTING TO FLOOR LEVEL

The patient sits on a low stool, 20–25 cm high, with the legs stretched out in front of him and with the heels resting on the floor; the hands grasp the sides of the stool (low grasp inclined long sitting) (*Fig.* 39*a*). Taking the weight on his hands he eases the pelvis slightly forwards and lowers it on to the floor with the trunk held erect (*Fig.* 39*b*). During this manœuvre the knees and hips are well flexed, and the main muscle work is confined to the extensors of the elbows.

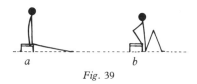

*Fig.* 39

From the position shown in *Fig.* 39*b* the legs are then straightened out and the palms of the hands placed on the floor (long sitting).

*N.B.* The use of a stool or chair higher than that recommended prohibits the use of this manœuvre because of the demands made on the working muscles and the stresses imposed on the shoulder joints and shoulder girdle.

## MOVING FROM STANDING TO FLOOR LEVEL

### Hands Supported on Chair Seat

The patient faces the front of a chair seat with his feet about a foot-length away from the front edge. He places the palms of the hands flat on the seat so that the trunk assumes a horizontal position. He then carries one leg backwards and places the foot on the floor with the ankle dorsiflexed (*Fig.* 40*a*).

The body is lowered downwards until the patient is in a modified half kneeling position (*Fig.* 40*b*). The forward leg is then carried back until it lies alongside the other; this brings the patient into the kneeling position with the palms of the hands resting on the chair seat (*Fig.* 40*c*).

From this position the patient places the right hand on the floor, just lateral to the right knee. The body is then lowered sideways in the direction of the hand to assume a right side sitting position (p. 267), with the left hand still resting on the chair seat. This hand is then placed on the floor by the side of the left lower leg.

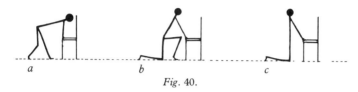

*Fig.* 40.

From side sitting a variety of other positions may be readily assumed: long sitting, crook sitting, crook side-lying, prone kneeling and prone lying.

N.B. The back of a chair can also be used to give support during the body lowering (*see below*). It is less stable than the chair seat but has the advantage of allowing the patient to keep the spine erect during the initial stages of the movement.

## Hands Grasping Chair Back

The patient grasps the back of a chair (which must have a stable base) with the body positioned as shown in *Fig.* 41*a*. The arms are shoulder-width apart and the weight of the rear leg rests on the toes.

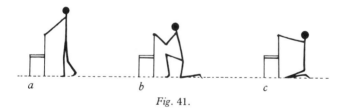

*Fig.* 41.

Taking most of the body weight on the hands the patient lowers the body to a modified half-kneeling position (*Fig.* 41*b*). He then moves the forward leg backwards until he is in the kneeling position with the hands still holding the chair back. The pelvis is then lowered backwards until the buttocks rest on the heels (*Fig.* 41*c*).

The right hand is taken off the chair back and placed on the floor, just lateral to the right knee. The body is lowered sideways in the direction of the hand to assume a right-side sitting position (p. 267), with the left hand still holding the chair back to provide a steadying effect. This hand is then placed on the floor by the side of the left lower leg.

From side sitting many other positions may be assumed, as outlined in the previous section.

## MOVING FROM SITTING TO STANDING

### Sitting in Chair with Arms

From the sitting position the patient places the hands well forward on the chair arms and draws the heels slightly back to bring them underneath the front edge of the chair. The hands then grip the chair arms and the trunk is inclined slightly forwards (*Fig.* 42*a*). The elbows are now extended and at the same time extension of the hips and knees takes place, the inclined position of the trunk being maintained. During this movement the hands take the weight of the trunk (*Fig.* 42*b*).

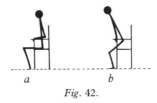

a                              b

*Fig.* 42.

When the body weight is fully over the feet (by continuous extension of hips and knees) the hands are removed from the chair and the arms are allowed to hang loosely at the sides. The patient is then in standing.

*N.B.* For the elderly and the disabled chairs with arms are essential. They can then help themselves to stand by using their hands and arms, as previously described. The base of the chair should be as wide and stable as possible to prevent tipping when the patient endeavours to stand.

### Sitting in Chair without Arms

Moving from sitting to standing is achieved in much the same manner as previously described, but the patient starts by having the palms of the hands resting over the lower thighs. In rising he exerts downward pressure on the thighs.

For the elderly and the disabled getting up from a chair without arms can be a somewhat precarious manœuvre. Much depends on the physical ability of the individual concerned.

### Sitting over Side of Bed

To achieve standing from this position the height of the bed must allow the patient to sit comfortably with the thighs fully supported, the feet resting flat on the floor, and the knees flexed to a right angle.

The actual rising technique is the same as described in the previous section (Sitting in Chair with Arms), but the patient's hands either rest on the mattress or are placed over the lower third of the thighs. Handgrips mounted on rectangular-shaped boards (*see Fig.* 33, p. 48) may be used to prevent the hands sinking into the mattress as downward pressure is exerted.

*Use of Chair*

The rising movements can be aided by positioning a chair with arms at the head of the bed, as shown in *Fig.* 43. In getting up from the bed the patient presses down strongly on the mattress with one hand, and grasps the chair arm nearest to him with the other, so as to gain additional support.

*Fig.* 43.

*N.B.* With the patient standing with one hand holding the chair arm it requires the minimum of effort to manœuvre the feet and body through 90°, so that he comes to stand with his back towards the front edge of the chair. (During this re-positioning he has to transfer his grasp on one chair arm to the other.) The patient can now assume a sitting position, using both hands to assist in the lowering process.

## NEGOTIATING STAIRS—PREPARATORY METHOD*

### Ascending Stairs

The patient stands on the floor facing the stairs with one hand holding the banister rail; the toes are close to the riser of the first step.

To ascend the stairs the sound leg is raised and the sole of the foot placed well forwards on the first tread by flexion of hip and knee. (During this movement weight is taken on the affected leg, and the hand on the banister provides additional support.) (*Fig.* 44*a*.) The body is then inclined slightly forwards, the weight being taken principally by the flexed sound limb, while the hand on the banister continues to provide support.

The sound limb is then straightened fully and the trunk raised to the erect position. At the same time the weak leg is lifted (flexed slightly at hip and knee) and the foot placed on the first tread alongside the other foot (*Fig.* 44*b*).

The same stair-climbing technique is used to negotiate the rest of the stairs.

---

*\* Preparatory Method.* The simple method of negotiating stairs described here is used when the weakness of one leg prevents the patient moving up and down stairs in a normal manner. The same basic pattern is followed when sticks or crutches are used and full weight-bearing on the weak leg is not allowed. The methods of using these aids in stair work are outside the scope of this section and have not been described.

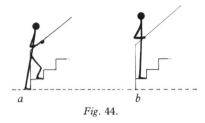

Fig. 44.

Ideally, to achieve maximum support—although this is often not a practicable proposition—the banister should be on the side of the affected leg.

## Descending Stairs

The patient stands at the head of the stairs with the toes close to the edge; he holds the banister rail with one hand.

To descend the stairs the weight of the body is taken on the sound leg, and the weak leg is carried forwards so that the back of the heel is close to the top of the first riser. The hand on the banister provides support during this movement (*Fig.* 45).

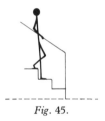

Fig. 45.

The body is then lowered downwards, by controlled flexion of the hip and knee of the sound leg, and the foot of the weak leg is placed on the first stair tread. The weak leg is now straight and fully extended at the knee. (*During this stage it is advisable for the patient to incline the body backwards a few degrees to counteract any tendency to tip forwards.*)

Full body weight is then transferred to the weak leg, with the hand on the banister offering support, and the trunk is held erect.

Next, the flexed sound leg is carried forwards, extended, and the foot placed alongside the other foot on the stair tread.

The same leg-placing technique is used to negotiate the rest of the stairs.

# PART 3

# PROGRESSIVE EXERCISES

## Introduction

The free exercises listed here are arranged progressively in terms of strength and mobility, as described in Chapter 2 (pp. 7–12), and include movements for all parts of the body.

In arranging the neck and trunk exercises, where a wide range of exercises has to be covered, each section devoted to a particular muscle group is divided into *Static* or *Isometric Exercises* and *Dynamic* or *Isotonic Exercises*, together with a brief analysis of the main type of movement.

*Grading.* All the exercises listed are grouped under three main headings: *Early*, *Intermediate* and *Advanced*. In turn, each group is divided, whenever feasible, into two or more grades.

Numbers prefixing the exercises indicate progression throughout the various grades. Where more than one exercise of the same type is listed in a grade, the number is followed by a, b or c to indicate this. *See* p. 82, Intermediate Exercises for Spinal Extensors.

# 7. Head and neck exercises

Head and neck exercises provide work for the muscles which activate the atlanto-occipital joints and the joints of the cervical spine. The exercises given here have been classified in relation to the individual muscle groups.

*Starting Positions*
Many types of starting positions are used for head and neck exercises, but those most useful for remedial work are sitting, low grasp sitting (*Fig.* 46) and reach grasp sitting (*Fig.* 47). Crook sitting and cross sitting (*Figs.* 48 and 49) are often used in the treatment of small children. The low grasp and reach grasp sitting positions are valuable when head side bending and head turning exercises are performed, because the shoulders are fixed.

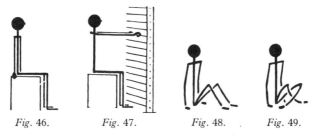

Fig. 46.     Fig. 47.     Fig. 48.     Fig. 49.

In this chapter the sitting position has been used when describing exercises which may be performed from it or any of its suitable modifications.

## FLEXORS OF HEAD AND NECK
### Types of Dynamic Exercises
*Head on Trunk*
Three main groups of exercises are classified here.

1. Flexion of the head and neck from lying and crook lying.
Example: *Yard (palms on floor) lying; Head bending forwards (Fig. 50).*
2. Part-range (from and to midline) extension and flexion of the head and neck from sitting.

Example: *Sitting; Head bending backwards.*

3. Full-range flexion and extension of the head and neck from the high lying position with the head unsupported.

Example: *High lying (plinth: head unsupported); Head bending forwards and backwards, and return to starting position (Fig. 51).*

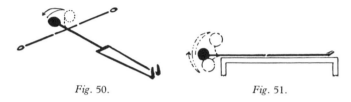

Fig. 50.                    Fig. 51.

## Strengthening Exercises

*Elementary*

GRADE 1

1. Sitting; Head bending backwards.

GRADE 2

1. No progression.
2. Yard (palms on floor) lying; Head bending forwards. (*See Fig. 50.*)

*Intermediate*

GRADE 1

1. No progression.
2. High lying (plinth: head unsupported); Head bending forwards and backwards, and return to starting position. (*See Fig. 51.*)

## EXTENSORS OF HEAD AND NECK

### Types of Static Exercises

1. *Attempted Movement*

Attempted movement of the head and neck from lying and crook lying without movement of the joints.

Example: *Lying; Head pressing backwards.*

2. *Fixation of Head and Neck*

Stabilization of the head and neck in the Body raising type of exercise from a suitable lying position.

Example: *Stride lying (head supported by partner); 'Log raising' by partner (Fig. 52).*

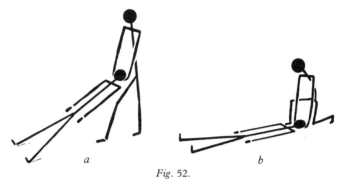

*Fig.* 52.

## Strengthening Exercises

*Elementary*: No. 1, p. 62; *Advanced*: No. 2, above.


## Types of Dynamic Exercises

1. *Head on Trunk*

Two main groups of exercises are classified here:

   *a.* Part-range (from and to midline) flexion and extension of the head and neck from sitting or extension of the head and neck from prone lying.

   Example: (i) *Sitting; Head bending forwards.*

           (ii) *Forehead rest prone lying; Head bending backwards.*

   *b.* Full-range flexion and extension of the head and neck from prone kneeling.

   Example: *Prone kneeling; Head bending forwards and backwards, and return to starting position (Fig. 53).*

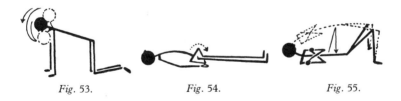

| *Fig.* 53. | *Fig.* 54. | *Fig.* 55. |


2. *Trunk on Head*

This group includes the Chest raising and Wrestler's Bridge types of exercises; they are performed from such starting positions as lying, crook lying, and stride crook lying.

   Examples: (i) *Lying; Chest raising (Fig. 54).*

            (ii) *Arm cross stride crook lying (head on mat); press up to high Wrestler's Bridge (Fig. 55).*

## Strengthening Exercises

*Elementary*

GRADE 1

1. Sitting; Head bending forwards.

GRADE 2

1. Prone kneeling; Head bending forwards and backwards, and return to starting position. (*See Fig.* 53, p. 63.)
2. Forehead rest prone lying; Head bending backwards.
3. Lying; Chest raising. (*See Fig.* 54, p. 63.)

*Intermediate*

GRADE 1

1 and 2. No progressions.
3. Crook lying; Chest raising.

GRADE 2

1 and 2. No progressions.
3. Neck rest crook lying; Chest raising.

*Advanced*

GRADE 1

1 and 2. No progressions.
3. Arm cross stride crook lying (head on mat); press up to high Wrestler's Bridge. (*See Fig.* 55, p. 63.)

GRADE 2

1 and 2. No progressions.
3. Arm cross stride lying (head on mat); press up to low Wrestler's Bridge (*Fig.* 56).

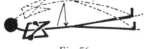

*Fig.* 56.

## Mobilizing Exercises

*Elementary*

GRADE 1

1. Sitting; Head dropping forwards and stretching upwards.
2. Sitting; Head nodding forwards (1–2), followed by stretching upwards (3–4).

GRADE 2

1. Prone kneeling; Head bending forwards, and bending backwards with rhythmical pressing to a given count, followed by return to starting position.

1a. Prone kneeling; Head bending forwards and backwards continuously.

2. Prone kneeling; Head dropping forwards and bending backwards.

3. Forehead rest prone lying; Head bending backwards with rhythmical pressing to a given count.


## FLEXORS AND EXTENSORS OF HEAD AND NECK

### Types of Dynamic Exercises

*Head on Trunk*

Three main groups of exercises are classified here.

1. Full-range flexion and extension of the head and neck from crook side-lying.

Example: *Crook side-lying; Head bending forwards and backwards, and return to starting position.*

2. Part-range (from and to midline) or full-range flexion and extension of the head and neck from sitting.

Example: *Sitting; Head bending forwards to press the chin gently against the chest, followed by Head bending backwards, and return to starting position.*

3. Straightening of the cervical concavity with slight flexion of the atlanto-occipital joints, followed by flexion of the neck with extension of the atlanto-occipital joints (Chin indrawing and poking forwards). The movements are usually taken from sitting.


### Strengthening Exercises

*Elementary*

GRADE 1

1. Crook side-lying; Head bending forwards and backwards, and return to starting position.


GRADE 2

1. No progression.

2. Sitting; Head bending forwards to press the chin gently against the chest, and Head stretching upwards.

3. Sitting; Head bending forwards to press the chin gently against the chest, followed by Head bending backwards, and return to starting position.

4. Sitting; Chin indrawing and poking forwards, and return to starting position.

## Mobilizing Exercises

*Elementary*

GRADE 1
1. Crook side-lying; Head bending forwards and backwards continuously.

GRADE 2
1. No progression.


## LATERAL FLEXORS OF HEAD AND NECK

### Types of Dynamic Exercises

*Head on Trunk*

Lateral flexion of the head and neck from lying, crook side-lying and sitting.
Examples: (i) *Crook lying; Head bending sideways.*
(ii) *Crook side-lying (head resting on pillow); Head bending sideways (Fig. 57).*
(iii) *Sitting; Head bending from side to side.*


## Strengthening Exercises

*Elementary*

GRADE 1
1. Crook lying; Head bending sideways.

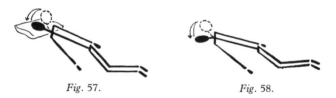

Fig. 57.                    Fig. 58.

GRADE 2
1. Sitting; Head bending sideways.


*Intermediate*

GRADE 1
1. Crook side-lying (head resting on pillow); Head bending sideways. (*See Fig. 57.*)

GRADE 2
1. Crook side-lying (head touching supporting surface); Head bending sideways (*Fig. 58*).

## Mobilizing Exercises

*Elementary*

GRADE 1

    1. Crook lying; Head bending from side to side.

GRADE 2

    1. Sitting; Head bending from side to side.

    2. Sitting; Head bending sideways with rhythmical pressing to a given count.

## ROTATORS OF HEAD AND NECK

### Types of Dynamic Exercises

*Head on Trunk*

Rotation of the head and neck from lying, crook lying, and sitting.

    Examples: (i) *Crook lying; Head turning.*

              (ii) *Sitting; Head turning from side to side.*

### Strengthening Exercises

*Elementary*

GRADE 1

    1. Crook lying; Head turning.

    1a. Sitting; Head turning.

### Mobilizing Exercises

*Elementary*

GRADE 1

    1. Crook lying; Head turning from side to side.

    1a. Sitting; Head turning from side to side.

GRADE 2

    1a. Sitting; Head turning with rhythmical pressing to a given count.

## CIRCUMDUCTORS OF HEAD AND NECK

### Types of Dynamic Exercises

*Head on Trunk*

Circumduction of the head and neck from sitting and prone kneeling.

## Mobilizing Exercises

*Elementary*

GRADE 1

    1. Sitting; Head rolling.

GRADE 2

    1. Prone kneeling; Head rolling.

# 8. Trunk exercises

Trunk exercises provide work for the spinal muscles which act on the thoracolumbar spine and pelvis; many of the exercises also activate the muscles of the hips, cervical spine and atlanto-occipital joints.

The exercises given here have been classified in relation to the individual muscle groups of the thoracolumbar spine.

## FLEXORS OF THE SPINE

### Types of Static Exercises

1. *Abdominal Retraction*

Retraction of the abdominal muscles from such starting positions as crook lying, prone lying, sitting and standing.

Example: *Crook lying; Abdominal contractions.*

2. *Leg or Legs on Trunk*

In this group of exercises the hips are flexed in turn, or together, through a given range of movement. The abdominal muscles act statically to prevent the pelvis from being tilted forwards by the contraction of the hip flexors of the moving leg or legs. When the legs are moved in turn the hip extensors of the resting leg act statically with the abdominal muscles to fix the pelvis.

Four main types of exercises are classified here. They are taken from such starting positions as lying, standing and hanging.

a. Flexion of the hip and knee of one leg almost to the full extent.*

Example: *Lying; single high Knee raising (Fig. 59).*

b. Flexion of one or both hips up to 90° with flexion of the knee or knees.

Example: *Lying; single Knee raising.*

c. Flexion of one hip through 45°, with the knee extended.

Example: *Lying; single Leg raising through 45°.*

---

* In the average subject flexion of one hip (with the knee well flexed) through the final degrees of movement is associated with small range backward tilting of the pelvis. Flexion of the hip should therefore not be taken to its full extent if a pure static action of the abdominal muscles is required.

*d.* Flexion of the hips to 45° with the knees extended.
Example: *Stretch grasp back towards standing (wall bars); Leg raising to 45°.*

3. *Trunk (Spine Straight) on Legs*

   *a.* Trunk lowering backwards and raising from fixed inclined long sitting with the spine held straight. The hips are alternately extended and flexed through a range of 35–65°.
   Example: *Wing fixed inclined long sitting (wall bar stool); Trunk lowering backwards through 45° (Fig. 60).*

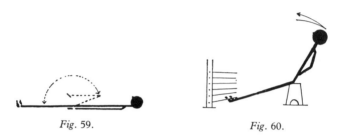

*Fig.* 59.                          *Fig.* 60.

During the raising and lowering movements the abdominal muscles act statically to maintain the straight position of the spine.
   *b.* Trunk raising and lowering from fixed lying or fixed crook lying with the spine held straight. The hips are alternately flexed and extended through a range of about 90°.
   Example: *Wing fixed crook lying; Trunk raising (Fig. 61).*
   During the raising and lowering movements the abdominal muscles act statically to maintain the straight position of the trunk.

4. *Head on Trunk*

Head bending forwards from lying and crook lying. The abdominal muscles act statically to fix the origin of the scalene muscles and the sternomastoid muscles.
   Example: *Crook lying; Head bending forwards.*
   Head bending forwards is often combined with hip flexion movements to increase the static action of the abdominal muscles.
   Example: *Lying; Head bending forwards with single high Knee raising.*

5. *Arm Bending from Prone Falling Position and its Modifications*

During the exercise the abdominal muscles act statically to prevent gravity from tilting the pelvis forwards and exaggerating the lumbar concavity.
   Example: *Inclined prone falling (hands on beam); Arm bending (Fig. 62).*

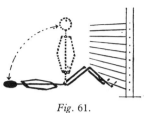

*Fig.* 61.

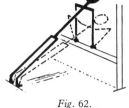

*Fig.* 62.

## Strengthening Exercises

*Elementary*

GRADE 1

1. Crook lying; Abdominal contractions.
2. Lying; single Knee raising.
3. Lying; single high Knee raising. (*See Fig.* 59, p. 70.)
4. Lying; single Leg raising to 45°.
5. Lying; single high Knee raising, Leg stretching forwards to 45°, and slow lowering.
6. Crook lying; Head bending forwards.
7. Lying; Head bending forwards with single high Knee raising.
8. Low grasp fixed inclined long sitting (hands grasping front edge of wall bar stool); Trunk lowering backwards through 35°.

GRADE 2

1. Prone lying; Abdominal contractions.
2. Lying; Knee raising (*Fig.* 63).
3. Lying; cycling.
4. Lying; alternate Leg raising through 45°.
4a. Lying; single Leg raising to 45°, followed by Leg raising to 15°.
5 and 6. No progressions.
7. Yard (palms on floor) lying; Head bending forwards with single Leg raising through 45°.
8. Wing fixed inclined long sitting (wall bar stool or balance bench); Trunk lowering backwards through 35°.
9. Inclined prone falling (hands on beam); Arm bending (*Fig.* 62).

*Intermediate*

GRADE 1

1. No progression.
2. Stretch grasp back towards standing (wall bars); Knee raising.
3. No progression.
4. Lying; Leg raising through 45°.

4a–7. No progressions.

8. Wing or fist bend fixed inclined long sitting (wall bar stool); Trunk lowering backwards through 45°. (*See Fig.* 60, p. 70.)

9. Inclined prone falling (hands on beam); Arm bending. (*See Fig.* 62, p. 71.)

GRADE 2

1–7. No progressions.

8. Wing or neck rest fixed inclined long sitting (wall bar stool); Trunk lowering backwards through 45–65° (*Fig.* 64).

8a. Wing fixed lying; Trunk raising. (*See Fig.* 61, p. 71.)

9. Prone falling; Arm bending (*Fig.* 65).

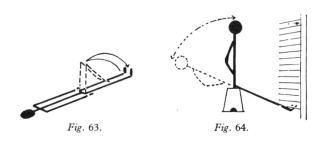

Fig. 63.                    Fig. 64.

*Advanced*

GRADE 1

1–7. No progressions.

8. Stretch fixed inclined long sitting (wall bar stool); Trunk lowering backwards through 45–65°.

8a. Neck rest fixed lying; Trunk raising.

9. Horizontal prone falling; Arm bending (*Fig.* 66).

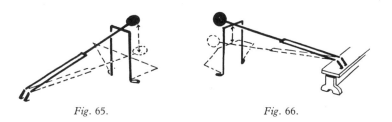

Fig. 65.                    Fig. 66.

GRADE 2

1–7. No progressions.

8. Stretch fixed crook sitting; Trunk lowering backwards to the floor.

8a. Stretch fixed lying; Trunk raising.

9. No progression.

## Types of Dynamic Exercises

1. *Spine on Pelvis*

Flexion of the spine without movements of the pelvis or legs.
Example: *Lying; upper Trunk bending forwards (Fig.* 67).

2. *Pelvis and Lumbar Spine on Upper Trunk and Legs*

Pelvis tilting backwards, the abdominal muscles acting with the hip extensors.
Example: *Crook lying; Pelvis tilting backwards (Fig.* 68).

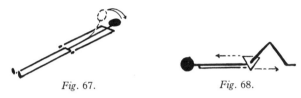

Fig. 67.                    Fig. 68.

3. *Legs on Pelvis: Pelvis and Lumbar Spine on Upper Trunk*

Full flexion of the hips and knees, or flexion of the hips with the knees extended, combined with flexion of the thoracolumbar spine.
Examples: (i) *Lying; high Knee raising (Fig.* 69).
(ii) *Lying; high Leg raising to touch the floor behind the head with the toes (Fig.* 70).

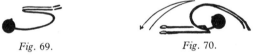

Fig. 69.                    Fig. 70.

A modification of this type of exercise consists of circling on rings or ropes. The extensors of the thoracolumbar spine work to a small extent, but the main emphasis of the exercise is on the abdominal and heaving muscles.
Example: *Stretch grasp standing (rings); circling and return circling with straight legs (Fig.* 71).

4. *Spine on Pelvis: Pelvis on Legs*

Flexion of the spine and hips, the legs being fixed by apparatus or living support.
Example: *Wing fixed crook lying; Trunk bending forwards (Fig.* 72).

5. *Combined Movements of Trunk and Leg or Legs*

Flexion of the spine combined with knee-raising movements; the legs are moved either together or one at a time.

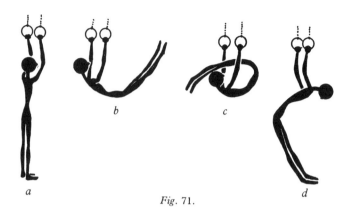

*Fig.* 71.

Examples:  (i) *Lying; high Knee raising, followed by over-pressure with the hands, and upper Trunk bending forwards (Fig. 73).*
(ii) *Lying; upper Trunk bending forwards with single high Knee raising.*

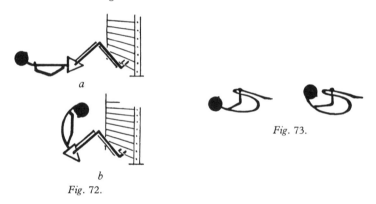

*Fig.* 72.

*Fig.* 73.

## Strengthening Exercises

*Elementary*

GRADE 1

1. Lying; upper Trunk bending forwards. (*See Fig.* 67, p. 73.)
2. Crook lying; Pelvis tilting backwards. (*See Fig.* 68, p. 73.)
2a. Crook side-lying (under hand grasping front edge of mattress, other hand pressing down on mattress in front of chest); Pelvis tilting backwards.

GRADE 2

1. Lying; upper Trunk bending forwards with single high Knee raising.
2. Prone kneeling; Pelvis tilting backwards.
2a. Reach grasp kneel sitting (wall bars); Pelvis tilting backwards.

2b. Reach grasp sitting (wall bars); Pelvis tilting backwards.

2c. Reach grasp standing (wall bars); Pelvis tilting backwards.

3. Lying; high Knee raising. (*See Fig.* 69, p. 73.)

*Intermediate*

GRADE 1

1. Fixed crook lying; Trunk bending forwards with assistance from the arms.

2–2c. No progressions.

3. Lying; high Knee raising, followed by overpressure with the hands, and upper Trunk bending forwards. (*See Fig.* 73, p. 74.)

GRADE 2

1. Wing fixed crook lying; Trunk bending forwards. (*See Fig.* 72, p. 74.)

2–2c. No progressions.

3. Lying (wall bars behind head); high Knee raising and stretching to touch a low bar with the toes.

4. Heave grasp walk forwards standing (rings); circling and return circling with bent knees, touching the floor with the feet at the end of the forward circling movement.* (*See Fig.* 71, p. 74.)

*Advanced*

GRADE 1

1. Neck rest fixed crook lying; Trunk bending forwards.

2–2c. No progressions.

3. Lying; high Leg raising to touch the floor behind the head with the toes. (*See Fig.* 70, p. 73.)

4. Heave grasp walk forwards standing (rings); circling and return circling with straight legs, touching the floor with the feet at the end of the forward circling movement.* (*See Fig.* 71, p. 74.)

5. Stretch grasp back towards standing (wall bars); high Knee raising.

GRADE 2

1–2c. No progressions.

3. Reach (or stretch) lying; high Leg raising to touch the floor behind the head with the toes. (*See Fig.* 3b, p. 9.)

4. Stretch grasp standing (rings); circling and return circling with straight legs. (*See Fig.* 71, p. 74.)

5. Hanging (wall bars); high Knee raising.

---

* The extensor muscles of the thoracolumbar spine act to a small extent, but the main emphasis of the exercise is on the abdominal muscles and the depressors of the arms.

GRADE 3

1–2c. No progressions.

3. Yard (palms on floor) lying; high Leg raising to touch the floor behind the head with the toes.

4. Inward grasp hanging (rings); circling and return circling with straight legs.★

5. Hanging (wall bars); high Leg raising.


## EXTENSORS OF THE SPINE

### Types of Static Exercises

#### 1. *Leg on Trunk*

Raising each leg backwards, in turn, from prone lying, so that the hip joint is extended about 15°. The extensors of the thoracolumbar spine and the hip flexors of the stationary leg act statically to prevent the pelvis from being tilted backwards by the contraction of the hip extensors of the moving leg.

Example: *Forehead rest prone lying; single slight Leg raising backwards.*

When hip extension is taken beyond 15° the pelvis tilts forwards, because of the tension exerted on the ilio-femoral ligament. The extensors of the thoracolumbar spine then act dynamically.


#### 2. *Trunk (Spine Straight) on Legs*

Trunk lowering and raising from such starting positions as sitting, stride standing, and fixed high thigh support across prone lying. The trunk is kept straight while the hips are alternately flexed and extended. The extensors of the thoracolumbar spine act statically throughout the lowering and raising movements to prevent gravity from flexing the spine.

The range of the hip movements varies in the different starting positions, as outlined below.

*a.* Sitting and stride sitting. The forward lowering movement is limited by the apposition of the soft structures of the thighs and abdomen.

Example: *Wing stride sitting; Trunk lowering forwards (Fig. 74).*

*b.* Standing and stride standing. The forward lowering movement is taken as far as the length of the hamstring muscles allows.

Example: *Wing stride standing; Trunk lowering forwards.*

*c.* Fixed high thigh support across prone lying. The position is usually taken over two balance benches, one being placed on top of the other. Trunk lowering forwards is limited by the contact of the head with the floor.

Example: *Wing fixed high thigh support across prone lying (balance benches, 2 high); Trunk lowering forwards (Fig. 75).*

---

★ The extensor muscles of the thoracolumbar spine act to a small extent, but the main emphasis of the exercise is on the abdominal muscles and the depressors of the arms.

This type of movement is usually introduced by a 'holding' exercise.
Example: *Wing fixed high thigh support across prone lying (balance benches, 2
high); position holding.*

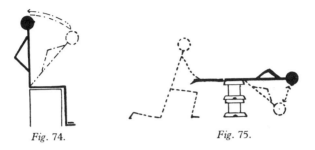

Fig. 74.                    Fig. 75.

### 3. Arm Bending from Fall Hanging Position or its Modifications

During the exercise the extensors of the thoracolumbar spine act statically
to maintain a straight position of the trunk and to prevent gravity from
flexing it.

  **Example:** *Over grasp fall hanging (beam at shoulder height); Arm bending
  (Fig. 76).*

### 4. Fallout Forward Exercises

The exercises are performed with or without arm movements. The extensors
of the thoracolumbar spine act statically to counteract gravity and to maintain
a straight position of the spine. Unless the exercises are performed with
perfect control the extensors will be used dynamically.

  Example: *Wing standing; fallout forwards, left Foot forwards, right Foot
  forwards (Fig. 77).*

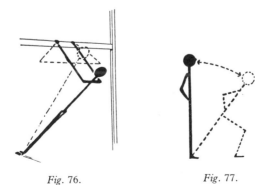

Fig. 76.                    Fig. 77.

## Strengthening Exercises

*Elementary*

GRADE 1

   1. Forehead rest prone lying; single slight Leg raising backwards.
   2. Wing stride sitting; Trunk lowering forwards. (*See Fig.* 74, p. 77.)
   3. Over grasp fall hanging (beam at shoulder height); Arm bending. (*See Fig.* 76.)

GRADE 2

   1. No progression.
   2. Wing stride standing; Trunk lowering forwards.
   3. Over grasp fall hanging (beam below shoulder height); Arm bending.

*Intermediate*

GRADE 1

   1. No progression.
   2. Fist bend stride standing; Trunk lowering forwards.
   2a. Wing fixed high thigh support across prone lying (balance benches, 2 high); position holding.
   3. Over grasp fall hanging (beam below shoulder height); Arm bending with single Leg raising.
   4. Wing standing; fallout forwards, left Foot forwards, right Foot forwards. (*See Fig.* 77.)

GRADE 2

   1. No progression.
   2. Neck rest stride standing; Trunk lowering forwards.
   2a. Wing fixed high thigh support across prone lying (balance benches, 2 high); Trunk lowering forwards. (*See Fig.* 75, p. 77.)
   3. Over grasp horizontal fall hanging (beam and living support); Arm bending (*Fig.* 78).
   4. Across bend standing; fallout forwards, left Foot forwards, right Foot forwards, with Arm flinging.

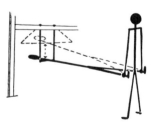

*Fig.* 78.

*Advanced*

GRADE 1

1. No progression.

2. Stretch stride standing; Trunk lowering forwards.

2a. Neck rest fixed high thigh support across prone lying (balance benches, 2 high); Trunk lowering forwards. (*See Fig.* 75, p. 77.)

3. Over grasp horizontal fall hanging (beam and balance benches, 2 high); Arm bending with single Leg raising.

4. Fist bend standing; fallout forwards, left Foot forwards, right Foot forwards, with Arm stretching forwards.

GRADE 2

1–4. No progressions.

## Types of Dynamic Exercises

1. *Pelvis and Lumbar Spine on Upper Trunk and Legs*

Pelvis tilting forwards, the extensors of the thoracolumbar spine acting with the flexors of the hips.

Example: *Crook lying; Pelvis tilting forwards (Fig. 79).*

2. *Leg on Pelvis: Pelvis and Lumbar Spine on Upper Trunk*

Raising in turn each leg backwards beyond 15° from prone lying or reach grasp standing. The ilio-femoral ligament of the moving hip joint checks hip extension after about 15°; to extend the leg further the pelvis is tilted forwards as far as possible by the extensors of the thoracolumbar spine and the flexors of the hip of the stationary leg.

Example: *Forehead rest prone lying; single Leg raising backwards.*

3. *Trunk (Spine Arched) on Legs*

This group includes Chest raising and preparatory Spanning exercises which are taken from lying and crook lying. The extensors of the thoracolumbar spine act with the flexors of the hips.

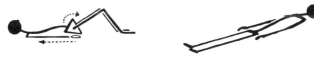

Fig. 79.                    Fig. 80.

Examples: (i) *Lying; Chest raising (Fig. 80).*

(ii) *High reach grasp lying (wall bars: hands grasping 5th or 6th bar from floor); spanning (Fig. 81).*

In these exercises crook lying is used as a progression on lying; it places the hip flexors in a shortened position, and so reduces their ability to raise the pelvis and lumbar spine from the floor.

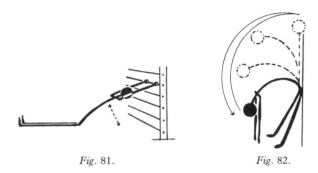

Fig. 81.                              Fig. 82.

### 4. *Spine on Pelvis: Pelvis on Legs*

In this group of exercises the extensors of the thoracolumbar spine are used with the extensors of the hips. There are three main types of exercises:

*a.* Extension of the spine and hips from lax stoop stride sitting or standing, or any other suitable starting position, to bring the trunk to the erect position.

Example: *Lax stoop back lean stride standing (heels 30–40 cm in front of wall or upright); Trunk stretching 'vertebra by vertebra' (Fig. 82).*

*b.* As the previous type of exercise, but the trunk is uncurled to the stoop position.

Example: *Fist bend lax stoop kneel sitting; Trunk stretching forwards to stoop position with Arm stretching sideways (Fig. 83).*

*c.* Extension of the thoracolumbar spine and hips from prone lying with the legs fixed.

Example: *Neck rest fixed prone lying; Trunk bending backwards (Fig. 84).*

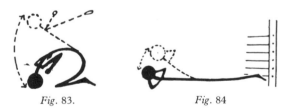

Fig. 83.                              Fig. 84

### 5. *Spine on Pelvis*

Extension of the thoracolumbar spine from prone lying. The extensors of the thoracolumbar spine are used dynamically; the extensors of the hips act statically to fix the pelvis.

Example: *Prone lying; Trunk bending backwards with Arm turning outwards (Fig. 85).*

### 6. Combined Movements of Legs or Leg on Pelvis with Extension of Spine

In these exercises the extensors of the thoracolumbar spine are used with the extensors of the hips. There are two main groups of exercises:

*a.* Spanning exercises and similar movements.

Examples: (i) *Angle hanging (wall bars); spanning (Fig. 86).*

(ii) *Arm cross stride crook lying (head on mat); press up to high Wrestler's Bridge. (See Fig. 55, p. 63.)*

*b.* Extension of the thoracolumbar spine from prone lying combined with extension of the lower limbs; the limbs are moved either in turn or together.

Examples: (i) *Prone lying; Trunk bending backwards with Arm turning outwards and single Leg raising backwards (Fig. 87).*

(ii) *Neck rest prone lying; Trunk bending backwards with Leg raising backwards.*

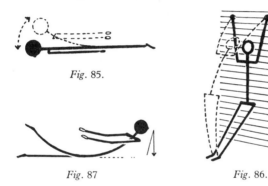

Fig. 85.

Fig. 87

Fig. 86.

## Strengthening Exercises

*Elementary*

GRADE 1

1. Lying; Chest raising. (*See Fig. 80, p. 79.*)

2. Crook lying; Pelvis tilting forwards. (*See Fig. 79, p. 79.*)

2a. Crook side-lying (under hand grasping front edge of mattress, other hand pressing down on mattress in front of chest); Pelvis tilting forwards.

3. Forehead rest prone lying; single Leg raising backwards.

4. Lax stoop stride sitting (hands on thighs, and lower part of sacrum in contact with wall or upright); Trunk stretching 'vertebra by vertebra' with assistance from arms.

5. Lax stoop kneel sitting (palms on floor with elbows bent); Trunk stretching forwards to stoop position with Elbow stretching.

GRADE 2

1. Crook lying; Chest raising.

2. Reach grasp kneel sitting (wall bars); Pelvis tilting forwards.

2a. Reach grasp sitting (wall bars); Pelvis tilting forwards.

2b. Reach grasp standing (wall bars); Pelvis tilting forwards.

3. Fixed prone lying; Trunk bending backwards with Arm turning outwards (*Fig.* 88).

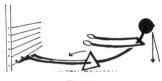

*Fig.* 88.

3a. Prone lying; Trunk bending backwards with Arm turning outwards. (*See Fig.* 85, p. 81.)

4. Lax stoop back lean stride standing (heels 30–40 cm in front of wall or upright); Trunk stretching 'vertebra by vertebra'. (*See Fig.* 82, p. 80.)

4a. Lax stoop kneel sitting (hands clasped behind back); Trunk stretching with unclasping of hands and Arm turning outwards.

5. As above, but Trunk is stretched forwards to stoop position.

6. Crook lying; Pelvis raising. (*See Fig.* 150, p. 116.)

*Intermediate*

GRADE 1

1. Neck rest crook lying; Chest raising.

1a. High reach grasp lying (wall bars: hands grasping 5th or 6th bar from floor); spanning. (*See Fig.* 81, p. 80.)

2. No progression.

3. Neck rest fixed prone lying; Trunk bending backwards. (*See Fig.* 84, p. 80.)

3a. Neck rest prone lying; Trunk bending backwards.

3b. Prone lying; Trunk bending backwards with Arm turning outwards and single Leg raising backwards. (*See Fig.* 87, p. 81.)

4. As Exercise 4 above, but arms in neck rest.

4a. Neck rest lax stoop kneel sitting; Trunk stretching 'vertebra by vertebra'.

5. Fist bend lax stoop kneel sitting; Trunk stretching forwards to stoop position with Arm stretching sideways. (*See Fig.* 83, p. 80.)

6. No progression.

GRADE 2

1. No progression.

1a. High reach grasp crook lying (wall bars: hands grasping 5th or 6th bar from floor); spanning. (*See Fig.* 4a, p. 9.)

1b. Stretch grasp back support kneel sitting (wall bars); spanning (*Fig.* 89).

2. No progression.

3. Head rest fixed prone lying; Trunk bending backwards.

3a. Prone lying; Trunk bending backwards with Arm turning outwards and Leg raising backwards.

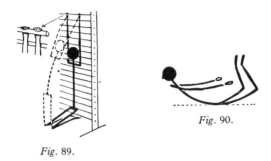

Fig. 89.

Fig. 90.

3b. Stride prone lying; Trunk bending backwards combined with Arm turning outwards, Knee bending and Leg raising backwards, so as to bring the heels together (*Fig.* 90).

3c. Prone kneeling; single Arm raising forwards-upwards with opposite Leg stretching and raising backwards (*Fig.* 91).

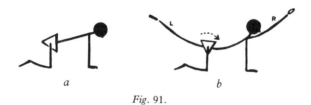

a                              b

Fig. 91.

4. No progression.

4a. Fist bend lax stoop leg backward stretch half kneel sitting; Trunk stretching to arch position (*Fig.* 92).

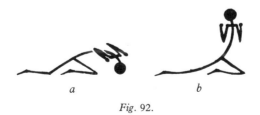

a                              b

Fig. 92.

5. Lax stoop stride standing (hands clasped behind neck, elbows forwards); Trunk stretching forwards with Elbow parting to neck rest position.

6. No progression.

*Advanced*

GRADE 1

1. No progression.

1a. Angle hanging (wall bars); spanning. (*See Fig.* 86, p. 81.)

1b–2. No progressions.

3. Stretch fixed prone lying; Trunk bending backwards.

3a. Neck rest prone lying; Trunk bending backwards with Leg raising backwards.

3b–4. No progressions.

4a. As Exercise 4a Intermediate, Grade 2, but arms in neck rest position. (*See Fig.* 92.)

5. Lax stoop stride standing; Trunk stretching forwards with Arm stretching forwards-upwards to stretch position.

6. Arm cross stride crook lying (head on mat); press up to high Wrestler's Bridge. (*See Fig.* 55, p. 63.)

7. Drag grasp lax stoop walk forwards standing (wall bars); assuming reverse hanging position (*Fig.* 93).

GRADE 2

1. No progression.

1a. Stretch grasp back support long sitting (wall bars); spanning (*Fig.* 94).

1b–2. No progressions.

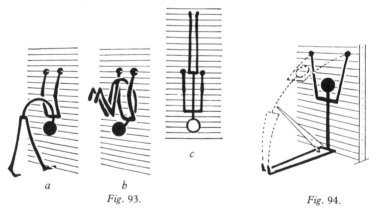

*a*                    *b*
*Fig.* 93.                              *Fig.* 94.

3. Neck rest lax stoop fixed high thigh support across prone lying (balance benches, 2 high); Trunk stretching to arch position (*Fig.* 95).

3a. Stretch prone lying; Trunk bending backwards with Leg raising backwards.

3b–4. No progressions.

4a. As Exercise 4a, Intermediate, Grade 2, but arms in stretch position. (*See Fig.* 92.)

5. No progression.

6. Arm cross stride lying (head on mat); press up to low Wrestler's Bridge. (*See Fig.* 56, p. 64.)

6a. Stride crook lying (palms on floor behind shoulders, elbows forwards); press up to the Crab (*Fig.* 96).

7. No progression.

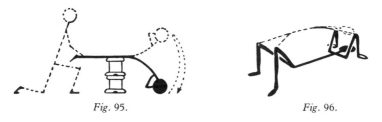

*Fig.* 95.                    *Fig.* 96.

## FLEXORS AND EXTENSORS OF THE SPINE

### Types of Static Exercises

*Trunk (Spine Straight) on Legs*

Combined movements of trunk lowering backwards and forwards (pp. 70 and 76) are taken from fixed inclined long sitting with the knees slightly flexed. The spinal flexors and extensors act statically to keep the spine straight, while the hips are alternately extended and flexed.

The backward lowering movements are taken through a range of 35–65°; the forward lowering movements are limited by the tension of the hamstring muscles. During trunk lowering backwards and raising, the spinal flexors are used statically; the spinal extensors act statically as the trunk is lowered forwards and raised.

Example: *Wing fixed inclined long sitting (wall bar stool); Trunk lowering backwards through 65°, raising and lowering forwards, and return to starting position (Fig.* 97).

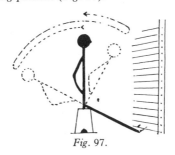

*Fig.* 97.

### Strengthening Exercises

Trunk lowering forwards movements are added to the trunk lowering backwards exercises which are performed from fixed inclined long sitting (pp. 71–72). *See* example above.

## Types of Dynamic Exercises

1. *Pelvis and Lumbar Spine on Upper Trunk and Legs*

Pelvis tilting forwards and backwards from such starting positions as crook lying, prone kneeling and reach grasp sitting. The extensors and flexors of the thoracolumbar spine act with the hip flexors and extensors.

Example: *Crook lying; Pelvis tilting forwards and backwards. (See Figs. 79 and 68, pp. 79 and 73.)*

2. *Combined Movements of Trunk and Leg or Legs*

a. *Simultaneous movement of trunk and each leg in turn.* The spine is flexed and extended in prone kneeling, the movements being accompanied by flexion and extension of each leg.

Example: *Prone kneeling; single high Knee raising with Head bending forwards, followed by Leg stretching and raising backwards with Head bending backwards, and return to starting position (Fig. 98).*

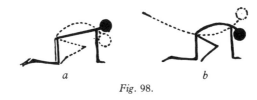

*Fig. 98.*

b. *Simultaneous movement of trunk and both legs.* This group of exercises includes:

i. Flexion and extension of the spine, hips, and knees in side-lying.

Example: *Side-lying; Trunk bending forwards with high Knee raising, followed by Trunk stretching backwards with Leg stretching and carrying backwards (Fig. 99).*

ii. Jumping the feet rhythmically backwards and forwards between crouch sitting and prone falling (*Fig. 100*).

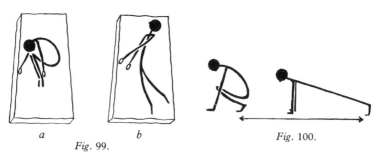

*Fig. 99.*     *Fig. 100.*

iii. Nest Hang exercises in rings.

Example: *Hanging from hands and feet (rings); Nest Hang (Fig. 101).*

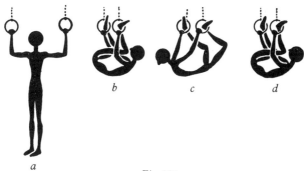

Fig. 101.

iv. Circling exercises at the beam.

Example: *Under grasp walk forwards standing (beam at head height); circling forwards-upwards and downwards-forwards with straight legs (Fig. 102).*

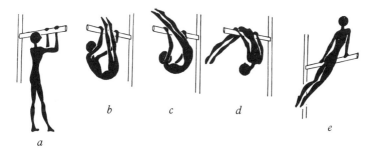

Fig. 102.

### 3. *Spine on Pelvis: Pelvis on Legs*

Two main groups of exercises are classified here:

a. Flexion and extension exercises of the spine and hips which incorporate rhythmical pressing or over-stressing movements in full flexion. The exercises are often considered to be of use in increasing flexion of the thoracolumbar spine and in 'stretching' the hamstring muscles. The usual starting positions for the movements are stride standing, long sitting, and fixed towards standing at the wall bars. (*See Fig.* 104, p. 88.)

Examples:   (i) *Stride standing; Trunk bending forwards-downwards with rhythmical pressing to beat the floor (1–3), followed by slow Trunk stretching upwards (4–6) (Fig. 103).*

    (ii) *Fist bend long sitting; Trunk bending forwards with Arm stretching forwards to reach the toes, or beyond them, with 3 presses.*

(iii) *Fixed toward standing (wall bars); Trunk bending forwards to grasp the ankle of the raised leg—over-stressing of Trunk bending—and slow stretching upwards (Fig. 104).*

All the rhythmical pressing and over-stressing trunk flexion exercises have been deliberately omitted from the list of mobility exercises in this section, because they are considered by orthopaedic surgeons to be wholly pernicious. *The exercises seldom do any good, and they are calculated to do the utmost harm to the spine, even when the hamstrings do not seriously limit hip flexion.*

A large number of people have congenital shortening of the hamstrings, and under no circumstances can these muscles be stretched. The force of attempting to stretch the muscles by spinal flexion exercises will be expended either upon the intervertebral discs, or upon the epiphyseal plates of the vertebral bodies. In the adolescent, damage to the epiphysial plates will be radiographically observed as osteochondritis, and the defective growth of the epiphysial plates may cause wedging of the vertebral bodies and permanent damage. In adults the force exerted on the fronts of the lower lumbar discs may be sufficient to rupture the annulus fibrosus of one of the discs and produce a frank prolapse of the nucleus pulposus.

*b.* Wide range *strengthening* exercises for the flexors and extensors of the spine and hips, which are taken from fixed inclined long sitting (*see Fig.* 105). The trunk is flexed to the *lax stoop* position, fully extended, and then returned to the erect position.

Example: *Wing fixed inclined long sitting (balance bench); Trunk bending forwards to lax stoop position, followed by Trunk stretching upwards, lowering, and bending backwards to touch the floor with the head, and return to starting position (Fig. 105).*

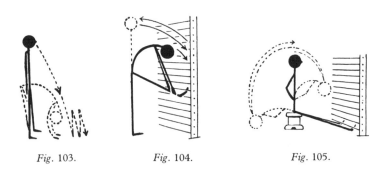

Fig. 103.                    Fig. 104.                         Fig. 105.

**Strengthening Exercises**

*Elementary*

GRADE 1

No exercises.

GRADE 2

1. Prone kneeling; single high Knee raising with Head bending forwards, followed by Leg stretching and raising backwards with Head bending backwards, and return to starting position. (*See Fig.* 98, p. 86.)

*Intermediate*

GRADE 1

1. No progression.

2. Under grasp walk forwards standing (beam at head height); circling forwards-upwards and downwards-forwards with bent knees.* (*See Fig.* 102, p. 87, which shows the exercise performed with straight knees.)

GRADE 2

1. No progression.

2. Under grasp walk-forwards standing (beam at head height); circling forwards-upwards and downwards-forwards with straight legs. (*See Fig.* 102, p. 87.)

3. Low grasp fixed inclined long sitting (balance bench); Trunk bending forwards to lax stoop position, followed by Trunk stretching upwards, lowering and bending backwards to touch the floor with the head, and return to starting position. (*See Fig.* 105, p. 88, which shows a different starting position.)

*Advanced*

GRADE 1

1. No progression.

2. Stretch under grasp standing (beam); circling forwards-upwards and downwards-forwards with straight legs. (*See Fig.* 102, p. 87, which shows an easier starting position.)

3. Wing fixed inclined long sitting (balance bench); Trunk bending forwards to lax stoop position, followed by Trunk stretching upwards, lowering and bending backwards to touch the floor with the head, and return to starting position. (*See Fig.* 105, p. 88.)

GRADE 2

1. No progression.

2. Under grasp hanging (beam); circling forwards-upwards and downwards-forwards with straight legs. (*See Fig.* 102, p. 87, which shows an easier starting position.)

3. As Exercise 3, Grade 1, but with arms in neck rest position.

---

* For introductory circling exercises at the beam, *see* Technical Points, p. 91.

## Mobilizing Exercises

*Elementary*

GRADE 1

1.  Crook lying; Pelvis tilting forwards and backwards. (*See Figs.* 79 and 68, pp. 79 and 73.)

1a. Crook side lying (under hand grasping front edge of mattress, other hand pressing down on mattress in front of chest); Pelvis tilting forwards and backwards.

2.  Side lying; Trunk bending forwards with high Knee raising, followed by Trunk bending backwards with Leg stretching and carrying backwards. (*See Fig.* 99, p. 86.)

2a. As the previous exercise, but during each trunk arching movement only one leg is carried back to the full extent.

GRADE 2

1. Prone kneeling; Pelvis tilting forwards and backwards with Head bending backwards and forwards (*Fig.* 106).

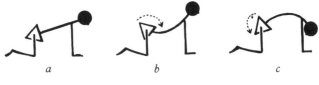

*a*          *b*          *c*

*Fig.* 106.

1a. Reach grasp kneel sitting (wall bars); Pelvis tilting forwards and backwards.

1b. Reach grasp sitting (wall bars); Pelvis tilting forwards and backwards.

1c. Reach grasp standing (wall bars); Pelvis tilting forwards and backwards.

2–2a. No progressions.

*Intermediate*

GRADE 1

1. Wide lax stretch (palms downwards) lax stoop kneel sitting; Pluto sniffing (*Fig.* 107).

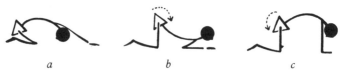

*a*          *b*          *c*

*Fig.* 107.

2–2a. No progressions.

3. Hanging from hands and feet (rings or ropes); Nest Hang. (*See Fig.* 101, p. 87.)

4. Crouch sitting; alternating between prone falling and crouch sitting by jumping the Feet rhythmically backwards and forwards (1–6). (*See Fig.* 100, p. 86.)

GRADE 2

1–2a. No progressions.

3. Hanging from hands and feet (rings); Nest Hang with single Leg raising backwards (*Fig.* 108).

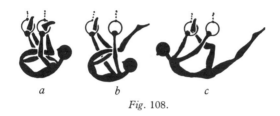

*a*　　　　*b*　　　　*c*

*Fig.* 108.

*Advanced*

GRADE 1

1–2a. No progressions.

3. Hanging from hands and feet (rings); half Nest Hang (*Fig.* 109).

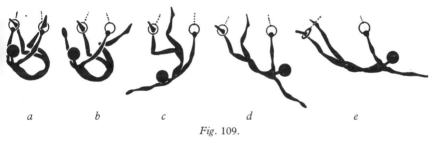

*a*　　　　*b*　　　　*c*　　　　*d*　　　　*e*

*Fig.* 109.

## TECHNICAL POINTS

### Introductory Exercises to Circling on the Beam

1. *Beam arranged at Hip Level*

The subject takes up an under grasp full squat position, with knees forward, so that the chest is pressed against the beam and the feet are under it. He then practises throwing the legs up to the beam with bent knees. Later, he attempts to straighten the knees and pull over the beam to the standing position on the other side.

## 2. *Beam a little under Hip Height*

The subject stands close to the beam, and grasps it with the fingers behind and the thumbs in front, so that the hands touch the thighs. He then leans over the beam as far as possible, simultaneously bringing the chin on to the chest and looking at the knees; he then bends the knees and brings the heels up to the seat, which allows the weight of the upper part of the body to carry the legs over the beam. The body should be kept in this curled-up position until the feet touch the floor.

## 3. *Using Two Beams: Lower Beam placed at Chest Level, and Upper Beam about 60 cm above it*

The subject takes up the under grasp walk forwards standing position at the lower beam. He throws the legs up and gets the heels behind the upper beam; he then presses with the heels and bends the arms and circles up on the lower beam to the balance hanging position (*Fig.* 243, p. 271). In circling forwards-downwards he bends the hip and knee joints as much as possible.

### Use of Supporters

Until the subject has acquired a good circling technique two supporters should stand on either side of him to give him confidence. Support is most often required when the subject changes his grasp before extending the body, and the assistants' hands should be placed under the shoulders and legs. It is also a wise precaution to put an agility mattress or mat under the beam in case the subject should accidentally lose his grasp.

## LATERAL FLEXORS OF THE SPINE

### Types of Static Exercises

#### 1. *Trunk (Spine Straight) on Leg*

Trunk lowering and raising sideways from standing or thigh support side towards standing by abducting and adducting the hip joint of one leg, the other leg being raised and lowered sideways with the trunk. Throughout the exercise the lateral flexors of the spine on the upper side act statically to keep the spine straight and to prevent gravity from side flexing it.

> Example: *Side toward standing (wall bar stool); Trunk lowering sideways to place the hand on the stool with single Leg raising sideways (Fig. 110).*

#### 2. *Lateral Movements of the Arm and/or Leg from Side Falling Position or its Modifications*

During the exercises the lateral flexors of the thoracolumbar spine on the lower side act statically to keep the trunk straight and to prevent it from sagging.

Example: *Side falling; single Leg raising sideways (Fig. 111).*

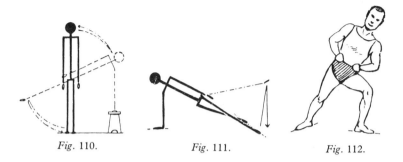

Fig. 110.          Fig. 111.          Fig. 112.

### 3. *Fallout Outward Exercises*

The exercises are performed with or without arm movements. The lateral flexors of the thoracolumbar spine of the upper side act statically to keep the spine straight and to prevent it from bending towards the side of the forward leg. Unless the exercises are performed with perfect control the lateral flexors will be used dynamically.

Example: *Wing standing; fallout outwards, left and right (Fig. 112).*

## Strengthening Exercises

### *Elementary*

GRADE 1

1. Side toward standing (wall bar stool); Trunk lowering sideways to place the hand on the stool with single Leg raising sideways. (*See Fig.* 110.)

2. Inclined side falling (hand on wall bar stool); single Leg raising sideways.

GRADE 2

1. Half stretch side toward standing (wall bar stool); Trunk lowering sideways to place the free hand on the stool with single Leg raising sideways.

2. Side falling; single Leg raising sideways (*Fig.* 111).

### *Intermediate*

GRADE 1

1. Wing thigh support side toward standing (beam); Trunk lowering sideways with single Leg raising sideways (*Fig.* 113).

2. Half fist bend side falling; single Leg raising sideways with single Arm stretching sideways-upwards.

3. Wing standing; fallout outwards, left and right. (*See Fig.* 112, p. 93.)

4. Stretch grasp high toward toe standing (wall bars); assuming Star position (*Fig.* 114).

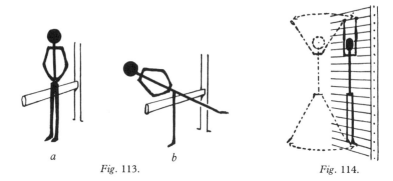

*a*               *b*

*Fig.* 113.                         *Fig.* 114.

GRADE 2

1. Half stretch half wing thigh support side towards standing (beam); Trunk lowering sideways with single Leg raising sideways.

2. Horizontal side falling; single Leg raising sideways (*Fig.* 115).

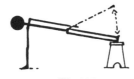

*Fig.* 115.

3. Fist bend standing; fallout outwards, left and right, with Arm stretching upwards.

4. No progression.

*Advanced*

GRADE 1

1. Stretch side toward standing (wall bars); Trunk lowering sideways to grasp the bars with single Leg raising sideways.

2. Half fist bend horizontal side falling; single Leg raising sideways with single Arm stretching sideways-upwards.

3–4. No progressions.

GRADE 2

No progressions.

## Types of Dynamic Exercises

1. *Spine on Pelvis*

Lateral flexion of the spine from a starting position which fixes the pelvis, such as ride sitting, stride sitting, and foot support side toward standing (*see* Fixation of Pelvis, p. 99).

Examples:  (i)  *Stride sitting; Trunk bending sideways.*

          (ii)  *Ride sitting (chair: thighs gripping chair back); Trunk bending from side to side (Fig. 116).*

        (iii)  *Half neck rest foot support side toward standing (wall bars); Trunk bending sideways towards the bars with rhythmical pressing to 3 counts (Fig. 117).*

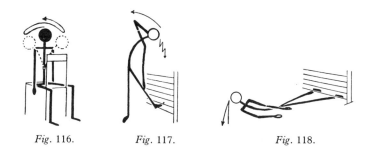

Fig. 116.          Fig. 117.                    Fig. 118.

2. *Spine on Pelvis: Pelvis on Legs*

Lateral flexion of the trunk from a starting position which allows lateral pelvic tilting to occur, such as stride standing, stride lying, and fixed side lying. The lateral flexors of the thoracolumbar spine act with the hip abductors and adductors.

Examples:  (i)  *Stride standing; Trunk bending from side to side.*

         (ii)  *Stride lying; Trunk bending sideways.*

       (iii)  *Fixed side-lying (one leg slightly in front of other); Trunk bending sideways (Fig. 118).*

3. *Legs on Pelvis: Pelvis and Lumbar Spine on Upper Trunk*

Leg raising sideways or leg swinging from side to side from hanging; this group of exercises includes leg lowering sideways from reverse hanging. The lateral flexors of the thoracolumbar spine act with the hip abductors and adductors.

Examples:  (i)  *Hanging (wall bars); Leg raising sideways (Fig. 119).*

        (ii)  *Over grasp hanging (beam); Arm walking sideways with Leg swinging from side to side (Fig. 120).*

4. *Pelvis and Lumbar Spine on Upper Trunk*

Hip updrawing from such starting positions as heave grasp lying and reach grasp standing. The pelvis is tilted sideways by the combined action of the lateral flexors of the thoracolumbar spine of the side of the raised hip, and the hip abductors of the opposite side.

Example: *Reach grasp standing (wall bars); Hip updrawing (Fig. 121).*

This group of exercises includes lateral pelvic tilting from side to side; the usual starting positions for these movements are reach grasp kneel sitting and reach grasp standing.

Example: *Reach grasp kneel sitting (wall bars); Pelvis tilting from side to side.*

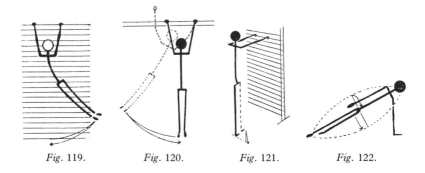

Fig. 119.          Fig. 120.          Fig. 121.          Fig. 122.

5. *Simultaneous Movement of Trunk and One Leg*

Lateral flexion of the spine combined with either *Hip updrawing* or *single Leg carrying sideways* of the side to which the trunk is moved. The movements are performed in lying.

Examples: (i) *Lying; Trunk bending sideways with Hip updrawing of the same side.*

(ii) *Lying; Trunk bending sideways with single Leg carrying to the same side.*

6. *Pelvis Lowering and Raising from Side Falling Position*

Pelvis lowering and raising from side falling by combined movements of lateral flexion of the thoracolumbar spine and hip abduction and adduction. The lateral flexors of the thoracolumbar spine on the underneath side of the trunk act with the hip abductors of the underneath leg and the hip adductors of the uppermost leg.

Example: *Side falling (one leg slightly in front of other); Pelvis lowering to touch supporting surface, raising as high as possible, and return to starting position (Fig. 122).*

## Strengthening Exercises

*Elementary*

GRADE 1

1. Stride lying; Trunk bending sideways.
2. Heave grasp lying (mattress) or lying (hands grasping sides of mattress); Hip updrawing. (*See Fig.* 121.)
3. Stride sitting; Trunk bending sideways.

GRADE 2

1. Lying; Trunk bending sideways with single Leg carrying to the same side.
1a. Lying; Trunk bending sideways with Hip updrawing of the same side.
2. Reach grasp standing (wall bars); Hip updrawing. (*See Fig.* 121.)
3. Neck rest stride sitting; Trunk bending sideways.
4. Neck rest stride standing; Trunk bending sideways.

*Intermediate*

GRADE 1

1 and 1a. No progressions.
2. Reach grasp high half standing (wall bars and stool); Hip sinking, updrawing, and lowering to starting position.
3. Stretch ride sitting (chair: thighs gripping chair back); Trunk bending sideways.
4. Stretch stride standing; Trunk bending sideways.

GRADE 2

1–4. No progressions.
5. Side falling (one leg slightly in front of other); Pelvis lowering to touch supporting surface, raising as high as possible, and return to starting position. (*See Fig.* 122, p. 96.)

*Advanced*

GRADE 1

1–5. No progressions.
6. Fixed side-lying (one leg slightly in front of other); Trunk bending sideways. (*See Fig.* 118, p. 95.)
7. Reverse hanging (wall bars); Leg lowering sideways (*Fig.* 123, p. 99.)*

---

* Leg lowering sideways from reverse hanging is easier for the working muscles than leg raising sideways from hanging. The reverse hanging position, however, is a difficult one for the average patient to maintain; for this reason leg raising sideways from hanging is often used before the other exercise.

GRADE 2

1–5. No progressions.

6. Half neck rest fixed side lying (one leg slightly in front of other); Trunk bending sideways.

7. Hanging (wall bars); Leg raising sideways. (*See Fig.* 119, p. 96.)*

## Mobilizing Exercises

*Elementary*

GRADE 1

1. Stride lying; Trunk bending from side to side.

GRADE 2

1. Stride standing; Trunk bending from side to side.

2. Ride sitting (chair: thighs gripping chair back); Trunk bending from side to side. (*See Fig.* 116, p. 95.)

3. Reach grasp kneel sitting (wall bars); Pelvis tilting from side to side.

*Intermediate*

GRADE 1

1. Neck rest stride standing; Trunk bending from side to side.

1a. Stride standing; Trunk bending from side to side with rhythmical pressing to 3 counts in position.

2. Neck rest ride sitting (chair: thighs gripping chair back); Trunk bending from side to side.

2a. Ride sitting (chair: thighs gripping chair back); Trunk bending from side to side with rhythmical pressing to 3 counts in position.

3. No progression.

4. Stride standing; Trunk bending sideways with single Arm (of opposite side) swinging forwards-downwards-sideways-upwards, the Trunk being bent to the side during the sideways-upwards swing of the arm.

5. Half neck rest foot support side toward standing (wall bars); Trunk bending sideways towards the bars with rhythmical pressing to a given count. (*See Fig.* 117, p. 95.)

6. Half neck rest leg sideways stretch half kneeling; Trunk bending sideways with rhythmical pressing to a given count (*Fig.* 124).

GRADE 2

1. Head rest stride standing; Trunk bending from side to side.

1a–4. No progressions.

---

* Leg lowering sideways from reverse hanging is easier for the working muscles than leg raising sideways from hanging. The reverse hanging position, however, is a difficult one for the average patient to maintain; for this reason leg raising sideways from hanging is often used before the other exercise.

5. Wing fixed side toward standing (wall bars); Trunk bending sideways towards the bars with rhythmical pressing to 3 counts, and bending away from the bars to 3 slow counts. (*See Fig.* 125, which shows arms in neck rest position.)

6. No progression.

7. Over grasp hanging (beam); Arm walking sideways with Leg swinging from side to side. (*See Fig.* 120, p. 96.)

*Advanced*

GRADE 1

1. Lax stretch stride standing; Trunk bending from side to side.

1a–4. No progressions.

5. As Exercise 5, Intermediate, Grade 2, but arms in neck rest (*Fig.* 125).

6. No progression.

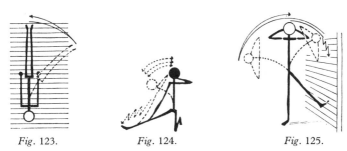

Fig. 123.          Fig. 124.          Fig. 125.

## Fixation of Pelvis during Lateral Flexion of Spine

The pelvis is securely fixed in the following positions:

1. *Ride sitting* on a chair, or a balance bench, with the thighs gripping the chair back, or the legs gripping the bench sides. (*See Fig.* 116, p. 95 and *Fig.* 126.)

2. *High ride sitting*, with the legs gripping the high plinth.

The pelvis is also firmly fixed in positions where one leg is supported, with the hips fully abducted; such positions include *foot support* (or *fixed*) *side toward standing*, and *leg sideways stretch half kneeling*. (*See Fig.* 117, p. 95 and *Fig.* 124.) The pelvis is less securely fixed in *stride sitting*.

## ROTATORS OF THE SPINE

### Types of Dynamic Exercises

1. *Spine on Pelvis*

Rotation of the spine from a starting position which fixes the pelvis, such as ride sitting and prone kneeling (*see* Fixation of Pelvis, p. 103).

Examples: (i) *Wing ride sitting (balance bench: legs gripping bench sides); Trunk turning (Fig. 126).*

(ii) *Prone kneeling; Trunk turning with single Arm swinging sideways and rhythmical pressing to 3 counts (Fig. 127).*

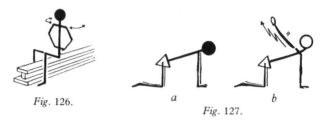

*Fig. 126.*        *a*               *b*

*Fig. 127.*

### 2. Legs, Pelvis, and Lumbar Spine on Upper Trunk

Rotation of the trunk by moving the pelvis and legs together, the upper trunk being the fixed point.

Example: *Yard (palms on floor) crook lying; Knee swinging from side to side (Fig. 128).*

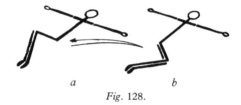

*a*            *b*

*Fig. 128.*

### 3. Spine on Pelvis: Pelvis on Legs

Rotation of the trunk from a starting position which allows hip rotation, such as stride standing, standing, and stride lying.

Example: *Stride standing; Trunk turning from side to side with Arm swinging loosely at the sides.*

### 4. Pelvis and Lumbar Spine on Upper Trunk and Legs

Pelvic rotation from a starting position which allows hip rotation and fixes the upper trunk and legs.

Example: *Reach grasp close standing (wall bars); Pelvis turning.*

## Strengthening Exercises

*Elementary*

GRADE 1

1. Wing ride sitting (balance bench: thighs gripping bench sides); Trunk turning (*Fig. 126*).

2. Wing stride-sitting; Trunk turning.
3. Stride-standing; Trunk turning.
4. Reach grasp close standing (wall bars); Pelvis turning.

GRADE 2

1 and 2. No progressions.

3. Stride lying; Trunk turning with single Arm carrying across the chest (*Fig.* 129).

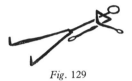

*Fig.* 129

4. Heave grasp lying (wall bars); Pelvis turning.
4a. Crook lying; Pelvis raising, turning, and lowering.
5. Prone kneeling; slow Trunk turning with single Arm raising sideways. (*See Fig.* 127, p. 100, which shows the movement performed as a mobility exercise.)

*Intermediate*

GRADE 1

1–4a. No progressions.

5. Turn prone kneeling (one arm bent loosely across chest); slow Trunk turning with single Arm raising sideways. (*See Fig.* 127, p. 100, which shows the movement performed as a mobility exercise.)

GRADE 2

1–5. No progressions.

6. Yard (palms on floor) half crook half vertical leg lift lying; Leg lowering sideways (*Fig.* 130).

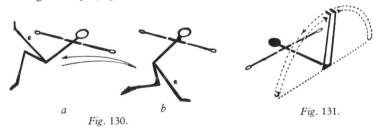

*a*        *b*        *Fig.* 131.

*Fig.* 130.

*Advanced*

GRADE 1

1–5. No progressions.

6. Yard (palms on floor) vertical leg lift lying; slow Leg swinging from side to side (*Fig.* 131).

## Mobilizing Exercises

*Elementary*

GRADE 1

1. Arm cross ride sitting (chair: thighs gripping chair back); Trunk turning from side to side.
2. Stride standing; Trunk turning from side to side with Arm swinging loosely at the sides.

GRADE 2

1. Across bend ride sitting (chair: thighs gripping chair back); Trunk turning from side to side with alternate Arm flinging.
2. Half lumbar rest stride standing; single Arm swinging forwards, and sideways with Trunk turning.
3. Yard (palms on floor) crook lying; Knee swinging from side to side. (*See Fig.* 128, p. 100.)
4. Prone kneeling; Trunk turning with single Arm swinging sideways. (*See Fig.* 127, p. 100, which shows a rhythmical pressing exercise.)

*Intermediate*

GRADE 1

1. Arm cross ride sitting (chair: thighs gripping chair back); Trunk turning from side to side with rhythmical pressing to 3 counts in position.
2. Stride standing; Trunk turning from side to side with Arm swinging loosely at the sides and rhythmical pressing to 3 counts in position.
3. No progression.
4. Turn prone kneeling (one arm bent loosely across chest); Trunk turning with single Arm swinging sideways and rhythmical pressing to 3 counts (*Fig.* 132).

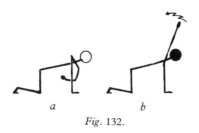

*a*      *b*

*Fig.* 132.

5. Reach half kneeling; Trunk turning with single Arm swinging sideways and rhythmical pressing to a given count.

GRADE 2

1–5. No progressions.

6. Over grasp fixed stride fall hanging (beam: feet fixed by living support); Trunk turning with single Arm swinging sideways to touch floor. (*See Fig. 134, which shows a more advanced exercise.*)

*Advanced*

GRADE 1

1–3. No progressions.

4. Lax reach stoop stride standing; Trunk turning from side to side with alternate Arm swinging sideways and across the chest (*Fig. 133*).

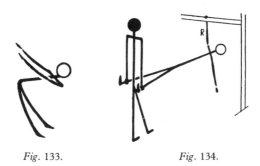

Fig. 133.                    Fig. 134.

5. No progression.

6. Over grasp horizontal fall hanging (beam and living support: beam at such a height that hand cannot touch floor if grasp of one hand is released); Trunk turning with single Arm swinging sideways (*Fig. 134*).

GRADE 2

No progressions.

## Fixation of Pelvis during Spinal Rotation

The pelvis is securely fixed in the following positions:

1. *Ride sitting* on a chair, or a balance bench, with the thighs gripping the chair back, or the legs gripping the bench sides. (*See Figs. 116 and 126, pp. 95 and 100.*)

2. *High ride sitting,* with the legs gripping the high plinth.

The pelvis is also well fixed in *prone kneeling (see Fig. 127, p. 100). Cross sitting* and *kneel sitting* give good fixation of the pelvis, but adults usually find these positions difficult to maintain. *Sitting, stride sitting, long sitting* and *crook sitting* provide some fixation of the pelvis.

## COMBINED EXERCISES FOR THE ROTATORS, FLEXORS, AND EXTENSORS

### Types of Dynamic Exercises

Only the main types of combined exercises have been classified here. All the exercises are based on the following sequence of movement—Spine on Pelvis: Pelvis on Legs.

1. *Working Flexors and Rotators of Spine with Hip Rotators*

Flexion and rotation of the trunk, without flexion of the hips, from lying and stride lying.

    Example: *Stride lying; upper Trunk bending forwards with turning and single Arm carrying across the chest (Fig. 135).*

2. *Working Flexors and Rotators of Spine and Hips*

Flexion and rotation of the spine and hips from fixed lying and fixed crook lying.

    Example: *Neck rest fixed crook lying; Trunk bending forwards with turning (Fig. 136).*

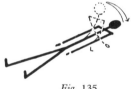 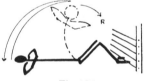

        *Fig.* 135.                       *Fig.* 136.

3. *Working Extensors and Rotators of Spine with Hip Extensors*

Extension and rotation of the spine, with extension of the hips, from a lax stoop position which prevents pelvic rotation. (*See* Fixation of Pelvis, p. 103.)

    Example: *Fist bend lax stoop kneel sitting; Trunk stretching 'vertebra by vertebra' with turning (Fig. 137).*

4. *Working Extensors and Rotators of Spine and Hips*

Extension and rotation of the spine and hips from such positions as fixed prone lying and lax stoop stride standing.

    Examples: (i) *Neck rest fixed prone lying; Trunk bending backwards with turning (Fig. 138).*

              (ii) *Lax stoop back lean stride standing (heels 30–40 cm in front of upright); Trunk stretching 'vertebra by vertebra' in different planes (Fig. 139).*

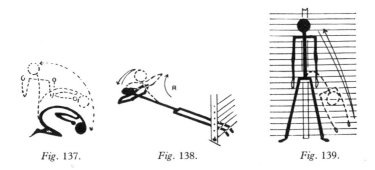

Fig. 137.            Fig. 138.            Fig. 139.

## Strengthening Exercises (Flexors and Rotators)

*Elementary*

GRADE 1

1. Stride lying; Trunk turning with Head bending forwards and single Arm carrying across the chest.

GRADE 2

1. Stride lying; upper Trunk bending forwards with turning and single Arm carrying across the chest. (*See Fig.* 135, p. 104.)

*Intermediate*

GRADE 1

1. No progression.
2. Fixed lying; Trunk bending forwards with turning, with assistance from arms.

GRADE 2

1. No progression.
2. Fixed slight crook lying; Trunk bending forwards with turning and single Arm carrying across the chest.

*Advanced*

GRADE 1

1. No progression.
2. Wing fixed crook lying; Trunk bending forwards with turning. (*See Fig.* 136, p. 104.)

GRADE 2

1. No progression.
2. Neck rest fixed crook lying; Trunk bending forwards with turning. (*Fig.* 136, p. 104.)

## Strengthening Exercises (Extensors and Rotators)

*Elementary*

GRADE 1

1. Fist bend lax stoop kneel sitting; Trunk stretching 'vertebra by vertebra' with turning. (*See Fig.* 137, p. 105.)

GRADE 2

1. As Exercise 1 above, but arms in neck rest.
2. Lax stoop back lean stride standing (heels 30–40 cm in front of upright); Trunk stretching 'vertebra by vertebra' in different planes (*See Fig.* 139, p. 105.)

*Intermediate*

GRADE 1

1. Across bend lax stoop kneel sitting; Trunk stretching 'vertebra by vertebra' with turning and single Arm stretching and raising midway-upwards.
2. As Exercise 2, Elementary, Grade 2, but arms in neck rest.

GRADE 2

1 and 2. No progressions.
3. Fixed prone lying; Trunk bending backwards with turning.

*Advanced*

GRADE 1

1 and 2. No progressions.
3. Wing fixed prone lying; Trunk bending backwards with turning.

GRADE 2

1 and 2. No progressions.
3. Neck rest fixed prone lying; Trunk bending backwards with turning. (*See Fig.* 138, p. 105.)
4. Wing lax stoop fixed high thigh support across prone lying (balance benches, 2 high); Trunk stretching with turning to arch turn position (*Fig.* 140).

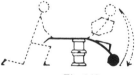

*Fig.* 140.

GRADE 3

1 and 2. No progressions.

3. Head rest fixed prone lying; Trunk bending backwards with turning. (*See Fig.* 138, p. 105.)

4. As Exercise 4, Advanced, Grade 2, but arms in neck rest position.

## CIRCUMDUCTORS OF THE SPINE

### Types of Dynamic Exercises

The exercises are based on the following sequence of movement—Spine on Pelvis: Pelvis on Legs.

1. *Working Circumductors of Spine with Hip Flexors and Extensors*

Circumduction of the spine combined with flexion and extension of the hips from such starting positions as ride sitting and high ride sitting.

Example: *Wing ride sitting (balance bench: legs gripping bench sides); Trunk rolling (Fig.* 141).

2. *Working Circumductors of Spine with Hip Muscles*

Circumduction of the spine combined with hip movements from stride standing and lax fall hanging (rings).

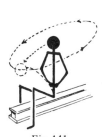

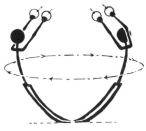

Fig. 141.                    Fig. 142.

Examples:  (i) *Wing stride standing; Trunk rolling.*
           (ii) *Lax fall hanging (rings); rolling (Fig.* 142).

### Mobilizing Exercises

*Elementary*

GRADE 1

1. Wing ride sitting (balance bench: legs gripping bench sides); Trunk rolling (*Fig.* 141).

2. Wing stride standing; Trunk rolling.

GRADE 2

1. Neck rest ride sitting (balance bench: legs gripping bench sides); Trunk rolling.

2. Neck rest stride standing; Trunk rolling.

*Intermediate*

GRADE 1

No progressions.

GRADE 2

1 and 2. No progressions.

3. Lax fall hanging (rings); rolling. (*See Fig.* 142, p. 107.)

## Strengthening Exercises

*See* Trunk rolling exercises in previous section. The movements are performed more slowly than when used as mobility exercises.

# 9. Breathing exercises

Breathing exercises may be divided into three main groups: (1) Bilateral or unilateral exercises which are localized to the respiratory muscles; (2) Arm exercises combined with breathing; and (3) Trunk exercises combined with breathing.

*Bilateral localized exercises* consist of Apical, Costal, and Diaphragmatic breathing, and General deep breathing. The best starting positions for these exercises are crook half-lying, crook lying and half-lying (p. 269). The respiratory movements are localized by the therapist's or patient's hands or by the use of a webbing strap or belt.

Examples: (i) *Crook half-lying (hands on sides of lower ribs); lower lateral Costal breathing with light pressure from hands (Fig. 143).*

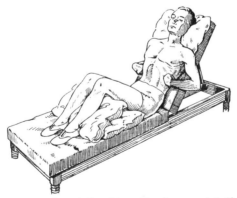

*Fig.* 143. Lower lateral Costal breathing from crook half-lying.

    (ii) *Crook half-lying (hand on upper abdomen); Diaphragmatic breathing, with emphasis on contraction of abdominal wall during expiration (Fig. 144).*

    (iii) *Crook half-lying (webbing strap round lower chest, with free ends held by hands); lower lateral Costal breathing with light pressure from strap (Fig. 145).*

Bilateral breathing exercises are used: (*a*) to increase the mobility of the thorax when the range of expiration or inspiration is reduced; (*b*) to ventilate

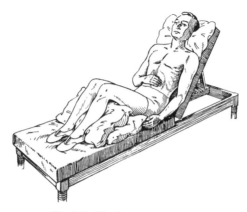

*Fig.* 144. Diaphragmatic breathing.

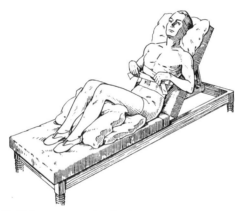

*Fig.* 145. Using a strap to localize lower lateral Costal breathing.

the lungs and prevent stagnation of mucous secretions; and (*c*) to teach correct breathing habits.

*Unilateral localized exercises* are used in the treatment of certain chest conditions. For example, *Crook half-lying (hand on side of left lower chest); left lower lateral Costal breathing with hand pressure (Fig.* 146), may be used in the treatment of empyema.

2. *Arm exercises with breathing*, e.g. *Stride sitting; Arm raising sideways-upwards with breathing.*

3. *Trunk exercises with breathing*, e.g. *Stride sitting; Trunk bending sideways with breathing.*

Physiotherapists tend to concentrate on the first group of exercises, because in the remainder the associated arm and trunk movements neutralize the action of the respiratory muscles; hence there is no net gain in respiratory

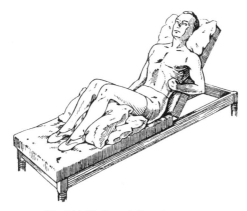

*Fig.* 146. Unilateral Costal breathing.

function. For example, in the exercise *Arm raising sideways-upwards with breathing* the ribs are fixed by the intercostal muscles, to stabilize the origin of the serratus anterior muscle; the fixation of the ribs neutralizes the upward dragging action of the pectoral muscles on the thorax, which would otherwise increase the range of inspiratory chest movement.

## BILATERAL LOCALIZED BREATHING EXERCISES

### Exercises to Increase the Expiratory Range

In these exercises emphasis is laid on prolonged, full expiration. Inspiration must be as easy and shallow as possible.

1. Crook half-lying (hand on upper abdomen); Diaphragmatic breathing with emphasis on contraction of abdominal wall during expiration. (*See Fig.* 144, p. 110.)

2. Crook half-lying (hands on sides of lower chest); lower lateral Costal breathing with pressure by hands on ribs during expiration. (*See Fig.* 143, p. 109.)

3. Crook half-lying (hands on sides of upper chest); upper lateral Costal breathing with pressure by hands on ribs during expiration.

4. Crook half-lying (forearms crossed and fingers resting on chest below clavicles); Apical breathing with pressure by fingers during expiration.

*In Exercises 1–3 a webbing strap may be used to localize the chest movements.* (*See Fig.* 145, p. 110.)

5. Slight stoop sitting (patient's forehead and arms supported on pillows resting on a table in front of his stool); posterior Basal breathing with pressure by therapist's hands during expiration. Alternatively, the patient may use a strap to localize the rib movements.

6. Crook half-lying; general deep breathing with emphasis on expiration.

7. Stride sitting; Trunk dropping loosely forwards–downwards to lax stoop position, with expiration, and Trunk stretching 'vertebra by vertebra' with shallow inspiration.

8. Stride sitting; Trunk turning with Arm swinging loosely at the sides: expiration during the backward turning movements, and shallow inspiration during the forward turning movements.

### Exercises to Increase the Inspiratory Range

In these exercises emphasis is laid on deep inspiration, followed by 'normal' expiration.

1. Crook half-lying (hand on upper abdomen); Diaphragmatic breathing with emphasis on the relaxation of the abdominal wall during inspiration. (*See Fig.* 144, p. 110.)

2. Crook half-lying (hands on sides of lower chest); lower lateral Costal breathing with light pressure from hands. (*See Fig.* 143, p. 109.)

3. Crook half-lying (hands on sides of upper chest); upper lateral Costal breathing with light pressure from hands.

4. Crook half-lying (forearms crossed and fingers resting on chest below clavicles); Apical breathing with light pressure from fingers.

*In Exercises 1–3 a webbing strap may be used to localize the chest movements and to give light resistance. (See Fig.* 145, p. 110.)

5. Crook half-lying; general deep breathing.

6. Skipping and rhythmical hopping exercises, running and swimming, to make the patient breathe deeply.

## EXERCISES TO VENTILATE THE LUNGS AND PREVENT STAGNATION OF MUCOUS SECRETIONS

The bilateral localized breathing exercises given in the previous lists are used, a full respiratory excursion being encouraged. Unilateral localized exercises are also used.

Postural drainage and some form of percussion, especially shakings and coarse vibrations, are frequently employed in association with the breathing exercises. The patient is also trained to cough effectively in order to assist the expectoration of the loosened secretions.

The coughing action is greatly improved if the therapist or the patient supports the sides of the lower chest firmly with the hands. Alternatively, support can be given by the use of a broad webbing strap, which is positioned as shown in *Fig.* 145, p. 110. The patient tightens the ends of the strap held in his hands to produce the necessary tension.

A Hawksley Cough-Lok (*Fig.* 147) is sometimes used in place of a webbing strap; it has the advantage of being about 10 cm wide and of being fitted with

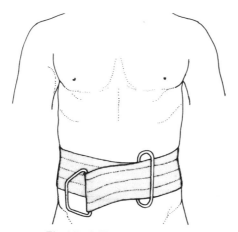

*Fig.* 147. A Hawksley Cough-Lok.

full-width Velcro fastenings. When adjusted in position round the lower ribs it provides the chest wall with an extremely firm and stable support.

Supporting the sides of the lower thorax in this manner during coughing has the effect of enhancing the upward pressure of the abdomen on the diaphragm and thoracic contents by preventing some of the pressure being expended in a lateral direction.

## TECHNICAL POINTS

### Practical Techniques

When the breathing exercises are first taught the therapist generally uses his hands to localize the movements for the patient. Later, when the patient understands the breathing techniques, he uses his hands or a webbing strap (about 1·5 m long and 7 cm wide) to localize the chest movements (*Figs.* 143–146, pp. 109 and 111). Light resistance may be given with the hands or the strap when the exercises are used to increase the range of inspiration.

When the therapist is localizing breathing movements for the patient, or supervising his breathing techniques, he should adopt a position which enables him both to feel and observe the respiratory movements without difficulty. The patient's head should be turned away from the therapist, particularly during expiration. This is not only in the interests of normal hygiene, but reduces the possibility of the therapist coming into contact with infected secretions.

### Starting Positions

Ideally, localized breathing exercises are carried out from a starting position which gives the body maximum support, relaxes the abdominal muscles, and does not require any unnecessary muscle work, e.g. crook half-lying (*Fig.* 143, p. 109), crook lying (*Fig.* 148) and half-lying. The head is generally supported by a pillow; in the crook and crook half-lying positions pillow support for the thighs is also very helpful in ensuring relaxation.

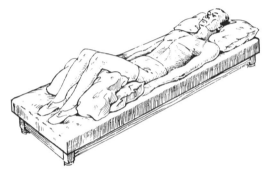

*Fig.* 148. Crook lying as a starting position for localized breathing: the thigh and head pillows ensure relaxation.

Other starting positions are used to achieve specific purposes. For example, a modified half-lying position (with the patient lying on one side) is useful in localizing movement to the ribs of the 'free' side. A modified stoop sitting position is also used for posterior basal breathing (p. 111).

*Physical Education*

From the standpoint of physical education sitting and standing may be used as starting positions for localized breathing exercises in addition to the positions previously described.

**Breathing Exercises in Physical Education**

Correct breathing habits are of considerable importance to the normal individual. For example, correct diaphragmatic breathing helps to prevent the development of lax abdominal muscles, and so indirectly assists in the maintenance of good posture. In the older age groups full diaphragmatic excursion is essential in order to ventilate the base of each lung adequately. Full ventilation prevents the accumulation of stagnant mucous secretions in the base of the lung, which are prone to become infected. Infected secretions may contribute to the formation of such conditions as bronchiectasis and lung abscess.

# 10. Pelvic floor exercises

Exercises to strengthen the pelvic floor muscles are used in the treatment of (1) Minor degrees of prolapse of the vaginal wall after childbirth, and (2) Stress incontinence caused by injury to the bladder sphincters, or, in women, by laxity of the muscles of the pelvic floor. Injury to the bladder sphincters may be produced by instrumentation or by prostatic resection.

Pelvic floor exercises are also used in ante- and post-natal training.

## TYPES OF PELVIC FLOOR EXERCISES

The muscles of the pelvic floor are exercised indirectly in three ways.

1. By contracting the hip adductors and the lower fibres of the gluteus maximus. This produces an associated contraction of the levator ani and the sphincters of the bladder.*

The hip adductors and extensors are exercised as separate groups or together from such starting positions as crook lying, lying, and standing. The muscles are also exercised in association with the sphincter ani.

Examples: (i) *Crook lying (soft pillow between knees); Knee closing.*
(ii) *Crook lying (soft pillow between knees); Knee closing with Pelvis raising and contraction of Sphincter ani.*

2. By activating 'the postural reflex between the abdominal wall and the pelvic floor whereby the pelvic floor contracts at the same time as the abdominal wall in order to withstand the strain of the increased intra-abdominal pressure'.*

The abdominal wall is exercised either alone or in association with the gluteus maximus and external sphincter ani from such starting positions as crook lying and crook side lying.

Examples: (i) *Crook lying (hand on upper abdomen); Diaphragmatic breathing with strong contraction of the Abdominal wall during expiration.* (*See Figs.* 144 and 148, pp. 110 and 114.)
(ii) *Crook lying (hand on upper abdomen); Diaphragmatic breathing with strong contraction of the Abdominal wall, plus Anal contraction, during expiration.*

---

* Yates-Bell J. G. and Cooksey F. S. (1937) *J. Chart. Soc. Massage Med. Gymn.* (Congress number: Sept.), pp. 28, 31, and 32.

(iii) *Crook lying; Pelvis tilting forwards and backwards, with emphasis on the backward tilting movement. (See Fig. 149, which shows a different starting position.)*

3. By contracting the external sphincter ani. It is possible that a contraction of this muscle is associated with a contraction of the pelvic floor muscles.

The external sphincter ani may be exercised independently or in association with the gluteal, abdominal, and hip adductor muscles. Specific exercises for the sphincter are performed from such starting positions as lying, crook lying, and standing.

Example: *Crook lying; Anal contractions (attempting to draw anus up into pelvis).*

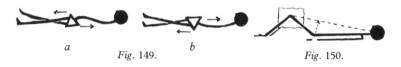

*a*          *b*
        *Fig.* 149.                    *Fig.* 150.

## Pelvic floor Exercises

*Elementary*

GRADE 1

1. Crook lying; Anal contractions (attempting to draw anus up into pelvis).

1a. As above, but with legs crossed. *Fig.* 149 shows the starting position.

2. Lying; Leg turning outwards with Anal contractions.

3. Crook lying (soft pillow between knees); Knee closing.

4. Crook lying (hand on upper abdomen); Diaphragmatic breathing with strong contraction of the abdominal wall during expiration. (*See Figs.* 144 and 148, pp. 110 and 114.)

5. Crook lying; Pelvis tilting forwards and backwards, with emphasis on the backward tilting movement. (*See Fig.* 149, which shows a different starting position.)

5a. As Exercise 5, but taken from crook side lying.

5b. As Exercise 5, but taken from lying, with legs crossed (*Fig.* 149).

GRADE 2

1 and 2. No progressions.

3. Crook lying (soft pillow between knees); Knee closing with Pelvis raising and Anal contractions (*Fig.* 150).

3a. Slight leg lift lying (legs crossed: heels supported on stool); Pelvis raising with Hip adduction.

3b. Inclined long sitting (ankles crossed); pressing Knees together with Gluteal and Anal contractions.

4. Crook lying (hand on upper abdomen); Diaphragmatic breathing with strong contraction of the abdominal wall, plus Anal contraction, during expiration.

5–5b. No progressions.

*Intermediate*

GRADE 1

1–3a. No progressions.

3b. Standing (legs crossed); Heel raising with Gluteal and Anal contraction.

4–5b. No progressions.

6. Walking while maintaining contraction of Gluteus maximus.

7. Standing; practising combined sustained Gluteal and Anal contraction.

8. Standing; practising coughing while maintaining combined sustained Gluteal and Anal contraction.

# 11. Shoulder girdle exercises

These exercises provide work for the muscles which activate the sternoclavicular and acromioclavicular joints *without* causing movements of the shoulder joint. Examples of some dynamic exercises are given here.

## ELEVATORS
### Strengthening
Sitting; Shoulder raising.

### Mobilizing
1. Sitting; continuous Shoulder raising and lowering.
2. Sitting; alternate Shoulder shrugging.

## DEPRESSORS
### Strengthening
1. Sitting; Shoulder depression.
2. Lying; Shoulder depression.

## ELEVATORS AND DEPRESSORS
### Strengthening
1. Lying; Shoulder raising and depression, and return to starting position.
2. Sitting; Shoulder raising, lowering, depression, and return to starting position.

## PROTRACTORS
### Strengthening
1. Sitting; Shoulder rounding
2. Lying; Shoulder rounding.

## RETRACTORS
### Strengthening
1. Sitting; Shoulder bracing.
2. Lying; Shoulder bracing.

## PROTRACTORS AND RETRACTORS
### Strengthening
1. Sitting; Shoulder rounding and bracing, and return to starting position.
2. Crook lying; exercise as above.

### Mobilizing
Sitting; Shoulder rounding and bracing.

## ELEVATORS, PROTRACTORS AND RETRACTORS
### Mobilizing
1. Sitting; Shoulder girdle rolling with emphasis on retraction.
2. As above, but with emphasis on protraction.

# 12. Combined shoulder joint and shoulder girdle exercises

In the majority of the exercises given here the shoulder girdle moves with the shoulder joint; in certain of the exercises, however, shoulder girdle movement is negligible, e.g. in rotation of the shoulder joint from the neutral position.

## 1. SHOULDER FLEXORS AND FORWARD ELEVATORS OF ARM

### Strengthening Exercises

*Elementary*

GRADE 1

   1. Bend lying; single or double Elbow raising forwards.

GRADE 2

   1. Bend sitting; single or double Elbow raising forwards or forwards-upwards.

   2. Bend sitting; single or double Arm stretching forwards-upwards.

GRADE 3

   1. Sitting; single or double Arm raising forwards or forwards-upwards.

   2. No progression.

*Intermediate*

GRADE 1

No progressions.

GRADE 2

   1. Grasp walk-forwards standing (stick crosswise in front of body); Arm raising forwards or forwards-upwards.*

---

  * *Stick Exercises*: The types of sticks used for these exercises are broomsticks and ash sticks. In general, broomsticks are more suitable for remedial work than ash sticks, because they are lighter.

120

2. Bend sitting (stick crosswise in front of chest); Arm stretching forwards-upwards.*

3. Grasp walk-forwards standing (stick crosswise in front of body); Arm bending, stretching forwards-upwards, and lowering to starting position.*

4. Reach grasp stoop stride standing (stick crosswise in front of body); Arm raising forwards-upwards.*

*Advanced*

GRADE 1

1. No progression.

2. First bend walk-forwards standing; single Arm punching forwards or forwards-upwards.

3–4. No progressions.

5. Grasp walk-forwards standing (Indian clubs); single Arm swinging forwards-upwards, and club circling backwards or forwards *behind* the forearm to 3 counts.

5a. As above, but both arms are moved together (*Fig.* 151).

6. Grasp walk-forwards standing (Indian clubs); single Arm swinging forwards-upwards, and club circling backwards or forwards *in front* of the forearm to 3 counts.

6a. As above, but both arms are moved together.

GRADE 2

1–4. No progressions.

5–6a. Grasp walk-forwards standing (Indian clubs); Arm swinging forwards-upwards, and club circling (*a*) backwards or forwards *behind* the forearms to 2 counts, and (*b*) backwards or forwards *in front* of the forearms to 2 counts. (*See Fig.* 151.)

## Mobilizing Exercises

*Elementary*

GRADE 1

1. Bend crook lying; alternate Elbow raising forwards.

GRADE 2

1. Bend sitting; alternate Elbow raising forwards.

---

* *See* footnote, p. 120.

GRADE 3

1. Crook lying; alternate Arm raising forwards.

2. Toward standing (wall); single (affected) Arm 'crawling up the wall' (*Fig.* 152).

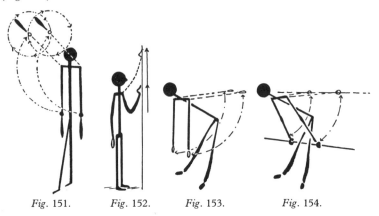

Fig. 151.        Fig. 152.        Fig. 153.        Fig. 154.

*Intermediate*

GRADE 1

1. Crook lying; alternate Arm swinging forwards.

2. No progression.

3. Walk-forwards standing; alternate Arm swinging forwards-upwards.

4. Walk-forwards standing; Arm swinging forwards-upwards, with increasing range to reach stretch position on the 4th count.

5. Walk-forwards standing; Arm swinging forwards and forwards-upwards.

GRADE 2

1–2. No progressions.

3. Walk-forwards standing; alternate Arm swinging forwards-upwards with rhythmical pressing to 3 counts.

4. Grasp walk–forwards standing (stick crosswise in front of body); Arm swinging forwards-upwards with or without rhythmical pressing.*

5. Grasp walk-forwards standing (stick crosswise in front of body); Arm swinging forwards and forwards-upwards.*

## 2. SHOULDER EXTENSORS

In these exercises movement of the shoulder girdle occurs after the shoulder joint has been extended fully. *See also* Exercises for the Depressors of the Arm, p. 127.

* *See* footnote, p. 120.

## Strengthening Exercises

*Elementary*

GRADE 1

    1. Bend sitting; single or double Elbow raising backwards.

GRADE 2

    1. Sitting; single or double Arm raising backwards.

*Intermediate*

GRADE 1

    1. Prone lying; single or double Arm raising backwards.

    2. Reach stoop stride standing; Arm raising backwards (*Fig.* 153).

GRADE 2

    1. No progression.

    2. Reach grasp stoop stride standing (stick crosswise behind legs); Arm raising backwards (*Fig.* 154).*

## 3. SHOULDER FLEXORS AND FORWARD ELEVATORS OF ARM WORKING WITH SHOULDER EXTENSORS

Many of the movements given in the previous sections may be combined (or the starting positions modified) to give wide range flexion and extension exercises of the shoulder joint, with movement of the shoulder girdle. Some examples are given below.

    1. Walk-forwards standing; alternate Arm swinging forwards-upwards and downwards-backwards.

    2. Half crook side-lying; single Arm swinging forwards-upwards and downwards-backwards.

    3. Reach stoop stride-standing; Arm raising forwards-upwards, lowering, and raising backwards as far as possible, and return to starting position.

## 4. SHOULDER ABDUCTORS AND SIDEWAYS ELEVATORS OF ARM

## Strengthening Exercises

*Elementary*

GRADE 1

    1. Sitting (affected upper limb resting on table, with shoulder abducted to about 90°, and elbow flexed); single Deltoid contractions.

---

* *See* footnote, p. 120.

GRADE 2

1. No progression.
2. Bend half-lying; single or double Elbow raising sideways.
3. Half crook side-lying; single Elbow raising sideways.

GRADE 3

1. No progression.
2. Bend sitting; single or double Elbow raising sideways.
3. Half crook side-lying; single Arm raising sideways (*Fig.* 155).

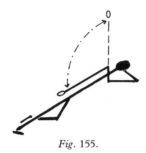

*Fig.* 155.

GRADE 4

1. No progression.
2. Half-lying or sitting; single or double Arm raising sideways-upwards.
3. No progression.
4. Bend sitting; single or double Arm stretching sideways-upwards.

*Intermediate*

GRADE 1

No progressions.

GRADE 2

1–3. No progressions.
4. Bend grasp stride standing (stick crosswise in front of chest); Arm stretching sideways-upwards.*

*Advanced*

GRADE 1

1–3. No progressions.
4. Fist bend stride standing; single Arm punching sideways or sideways-upwards.

---

* *See* footnote, p. 120.

5. Grasp stride standing (Indian clubs); single Arm swinging sideways-upwards, and club circling backwards or forwards *behind* the forearm to 3 counts.

5a. As No. 5, but both arms are moved together.

6. Grasp stride standing (Indian clubs); single Arm swinging sideways-upwards, and club circling backwards or forwards *in front* of the forearm to 3 counts.

6a. As No. 6, but both arms are moved together.

GRADE 2

1–4. No progressions.

5–6a. Grasp stride standing (Indian clubs); Arm swinging sideways-upwards, and club circling (*a*) backwards *behind* the forearms to 2 counts, and (*b*) backwards *in front* of the forearms to 2 counts.

## Mobilizing Exercises

*Elementary*

GRADE 1

1. Bend half-lying; alternate Elbow raising sideways.

GRADE 2

1. Bend sitting; alternate Elbow raising sideways.

2. Side toward standing (wall); single (affected) Arm 'crawling up the wall'. (*See Fig.* 152, p. 122, which shows the toward standing position.)

GRADE 3

1. Sitting; alternate Arm raising sideways-upwards.

2. No progression.

*Intermediate*

GRADE 1

1. Stride standing; Arm swinging sideways-upwards.

2. No progression.

3. Stride standing; Arm swinging to right and left, both arms moving in the same time and direction. (*See Fig.* 156, p. 126.)*

4. Low arm cross stride standing; Arm swinging sideways-upwards.*

5. Stride standing; Arm swinging sideways-upwards with increasing range to reach stretch position on the 4th count.

GRADE 2

1. Stride standing; Arm swinging sideways-upwards to beat the fists

---

* This exercise provides some work for the shoulder adductors.

together (1–2), and swinging downwards-sideways to beat the sides of the thighs (3–4).*

2. No progression.

3. Wide grasp stride standing (stick crosswise in front of body); Arm swinging to right and left (*Fig.* 156).†

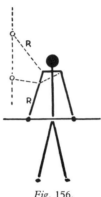

*Fig.* 156.

## 5. SHOULDER ADDUCTORS

In these exercises movement of the shoulder girdle accompanies movement of the shoulder joint. (*See also* Exercises for the Depressors of the Arm, p. 129.)

### Strengthening Exercises

*Elementary*

GRADE 1

1. Sitting (hands clasped in front of body with elbows flexed to about 90°); pressing palms together strongly to produce static contractions of pectoralis major.

1a. Sitting (hands and forearms resting on thighs); single or double Arm pressing inwards against the trunk to produce static contractions of pectoralis major.

GRADE 2

1 and 1a. No progressions.

2. Bend sitting; single Shoulder adduction, to move Elbow across the chest.

---

*This exercise provides some work for the shoulder adductors.

† *See* footnote, p. 120.

GRADE 3

1 and 1a. No progressions.

2. Sitting (elbows flexed to 90° and forearms in front of chest); single Shoulder adduction, to move Arm across the chest.

GRADE 4

1 and 1a. No progressions.

2. Stride standing; single or double Shoulder adduction, to move Arm(s) across the chest.

## 6. SHOULDER ABDUCTORS AND SIDEWAYS ELEVATORS OF ARM WORKING WITH SHOULDER ADDUCTORS

*See* Exercises marked with an asterisk in Section 4, pp. 123–126. Certain of the movements given in Sections 4 and 5 may be combined to give wide-range abduction and adduction exercises of the shoulder joint, with movement of the shoulder girdle.

## 7. DEPRESSORS OF ARM AND SHOULDER EXTENSORS

### Strengthening Exercises

*Elementary*

*See* Introductory Exercises to Arm bending from hanging, circling on the rings or ropes, and Rope climbing, pp. 129–130.

*Intermediate*

GRADE 1

1. Under grasp standing (beam slightly above head level); Arm bending with take-off from floor.

GRADE 2

1. Under grasp hanging (beam); Arm bending (*Fig.* 157).

2. Inward grasp hanging (beam); Arm bending (*Fig.* 158).

3. Heave grasp standing (rings or ropes); circling and return circling with bent knees, touching the floor with the feet at the end of the forward circling movement. (*See Fig.* 101*a*, p. 87, for starting position, and *Fig.* 71, p. 74, for exercise with straight legs.)

4. Under grasp walk-forwards standing (beam at head height); circling forwards-upwards and downwards-forwards with bent knees. (*See Fig.* 102, p. 87, which shows the exercise performed with straight legs.)

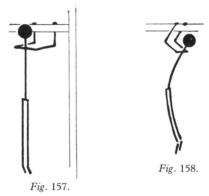

Fig. 158.

Fig. 157.

*Advanced*

GRADE 1

1–2. No progressions.

3. Heave grasp standing (rings or ropes); circling and return circling with straight legs, touching the floor with the feet at the end of the forward circling movement. (*See Fig.* 101*a*, p. 87, for starting position, and *Fig.* 71, p. 74, for movement.)

4. Under grasp walk-forwards standing (beam at head height); circling forwards-upwards and downwards-forwards with straight legs. (*See Fig.* 102, p. 87.)

5. Rope climbing: left or right Hand leading with Leg grasp.

GRADE 2

1–2. No progressions.

3. Stretch grasp standing (rings or ropes); circling and return circling with straight legs. (*See Fig.* 71, p. 74.)

4. Stretch under grasp standing (beam); circling forwards-upwards and downwards-forwards with straight legs. (*See Fig.* 102, p. 87, which shows an easier starting position.)

5. Rope climbing: Hand over Hand with Leg grasp.

GRADE 3

1–2. No progressions.

3. Inward grasp hanging (rings); circling and return circling with straight legs. (*See Fig.* 71, p. 74, for movement.)

4. Under grasp hanging (beam); circling forwards-upwards and downwards-forwards with straight legs. (*See Fig.* 102, p. 87, for movement.)

5. Rope climbing: Hand over Hand without Leg grasp.

## 8. DEPRESSORS OF ARM AND SHOULDER ADDUCTORS

### Strengthening Exercises

*Elementary*

*See below* Introductory Exercises to Arm bending from hanging.

   1. Stretch grasp high stoop standing (wall bars); Arm bending (*Fig.* 159).

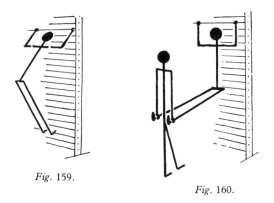

*Fig.* 159.

*Fig.* 160.

*Intermediate*

GRADE 1

   1. Angle hanging (wall bars and living support); Arm bending (*Fig.* 160).

   2. Over grasp standing (beam slightly above head level); Arm bending with take-off from floor.

GRADE 2

   1. No progression.

   2. Over grasp hanging (beam); Arm bending.

   3. Over grasp hanging (beam); Arm walking sideways with Leg swinging from side to side. (*See Fig.* 120, p. 96.)

### Introductory Exercises

*Arm Bending from Hanging*

*Subject Working with Partner.* The partner takes some of the subject's body-weight during the arm bending. He stands behind him, and grasps him at the waist.

*Exercise Performed from Standing.* The arm bending is performed from standing, with the beam arranged at stretch height. This allows the subject to rest his arms after each arm-bending movement.

*Circling on Rings or Ropes*

The subject attempts the circling in stages, first trying out a quarter turn, then a half circle, and finally a full circle. He need not attempt the return circle at first, but may let go of the rings or ropes and stand up when his feet touch the floor at the end of the forward circling.

Until the subject has acquired a good circling technique two supporters should stand on either side of him to give him confidence and, if necessary, to support him. It is also a wise precaution to put a mattress under the rings or ropes in case the subject accidentally loses his grasp.

*Circling on the Beam*

*See* p. 91.

*Rope Climbing*

*Leg Grip.* The subject practises taking and maintaining the leg grip, first with one foot behind the rope and then with the other. In the initial stages he sits on a stool which has been placed close to the rope. He grasps the rope as high as he can with both hands, and tries the leg grip without throwing any weight on to the arms. He must be taught to carry the feet well forward when he has gripped the rope, to prevent it from being held between the thighs instead of the knees; this would result in a weak grip.

The subject tests the grip by lifting his buttocks from the stool and swinging on the rope, or using his legs as in climbing. Thus he bends the arms and stretches the legs without losing his grip with the knees and feet, and then sits down on the stool again by allowing the arms to straighten out and the knees to bend.

*Ascending and Descending the Rope.* When the leg grip has been mastered the subject practises ascending and descending the rope from standing, without raising the hands much higher than stretch height. He then progresses to the full climb.

## 9. SHOULDER PROTRACTORS

Protraction of the shoulder joint 'is a movement in which the fully abducted arm is brought towards the fully flexed position'.* The movement is associated with protraction of the shoulder girdle.

---

*APPLETON A. B. (1946) *Surface and Radiological Anatomy*, 2nd ed., p. 46. Cambridge: Heffer.

## Strengthening Exercises

*Elementary*

GRADE 1

1. Neck rest lying; single or double Arm protraction.

GRADE 2

1. No progression.

GRADE 3

1. Yard (palms forwards) lying; single or double Arm protraction (*Fig.* 161).

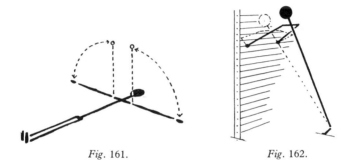

Fig. 161.                    Fig. 162.

*Intermediate*

GRADE 1

1. No progression.
2. Inclined prone falling (wall bars: hands between shoulder and hip height); Arm bending (*Fig.* 162).

GRADE 2

1. No progression.
2. Inclined prone falling (beam below hip height: hands supported); Arm bending. (*See Fig.* 62, p. 71.)

*Advanced*

GRADE 1

1. No progression.
2. Prone falling; Arm bending. (*See Fig.* 65, p. 72.)

GRADE 2

1. No progression.
2. Horizontal prone falling; Arm bending. (*See Fig.* 66, p. 72.)

## 10. SHOULDER RETRACTORS

Retraction of the shoulder joint is a movement in which the fully flexed arm is moved backwards through the horizontal plane to the fully abducted position. The movement is associated with retraction of the shoulder girdle.

### Strengthening Exercises

*Elementary*

GRADE 1

1. Neck rest (elbows forward) stoop stride standing; single or double Elbow parting.

GRADE 2

1. No progression.

GRADE 3

1. Reach stoop stride standing; single or double Arm parting.

*Intermediate*

GRADE 1

1. No progression.
2. Reach grasp stoop stride standing (stick crosswise in front of body); Arm bending to bring stick to chest (*Fig.* 163).*
3. Over grasp fall hanging (beam at shoulder height); Arm bending. (*See Fig.* 76, p. 77.)

GRADE 2

1–2. No progressions.
3. Over grasp fall hanging (beam below shoulder height); Arm bending.

GRADE 3

1–2. No progressions.
3. Over grasp horizontal fall hanging (beam and living support); Arm bending. (*See Fig.* 78, p. 78.)

## 11. SHOULDER PROTRACTORS AND RETRACTORS

For definition of protraction and retraction of the shoulder joint *see* previous sections.

---

* *See* footnote, p. 120.

## Strengthening Exercises

*Elementary*

GRADE 1

    1. Neck rest (elbows forwards) sitting; single or double Elbow parting.

GRADE 2

    1. Reach sitting; single or double Arm parting.

GRADE 3

    1. Yard (palms forwards) sitting; Arm carrying forwards to press the palms together strongly, followed by Arm carrying backwards to the full extent, and return to starting position.

*Intermediate*

GRADE 1

    1. Reach grasp walk-forwards standing (stick crosswise in front of chest); stick carrying backwards to the right, and return to starting position, and repetition of movement to the left.*
    2. Reach grasp walk-forwards standing (stick crosswise in front of chest); Arm bending in horizontal plane to bring stick to chest.*

GRADE 2

No progressions.

*Advanced*

GRADE 1

    1–2. No progressions.
    3. Fist bend stride standing; single Arm punching horizontally across the chest (*Fig.* 164).

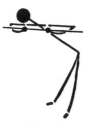

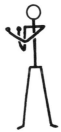

*Fig.* 163.        *Fig.* 164.

* *See* footnote, p. 120.

## Mobilizing Exercises

*Intermediate*

GRADE 1

1. Reach grasp walk forwards standing (stick crosswise in front of chest); stick swinging backwards and forwards in the horizontal plane.*

2. Across bend walk forwards standing; Elbow pressing backwards with Arm flinging on the 3rd count.

3. Standing (arms crossed firmly over chest); Cabman's warm-up swing.


## 12. LATERAL ROTATORS OF SHOULDER JOINT

### Strengthening Exercises

*See* Exercises in which the arms are raised sideways-upwards, p. 123. In these exercises the lateral rotators of the shoulder joint act with the shoulder abductors and the elevators of the arm.


*Elementary*

GRADE 1

1. Forearm reach sitting; single or double Arm turning outwards (*Fig.* 165).

2. Sitting; single or double Arm turning outwards.

GRADE 2

1. Forward heave lying; single or double Arm turning inwards through 90° (*Fig.* 166).

2. No progression.

GRADE 3

1. Half crook side-lying (elbow of uppermost arm flexed to 90°, and forearm in contact with chest); single Arm turning outwards.

2. Sitting; single or double Hand placing on back of neck or slight distance behind neck.


*Intermediate*

GRADE 1

1. No progression.

2. As Exercise 2, in previous grade, but performed in prone lying.

3. Heave grasp sitting (stick crosswise); Arm turning inwards to bring stick against chest. *Fig.* 167 shows the exercise taken from walk-forwards standing.*

---

* *See* footnote, p. 120.

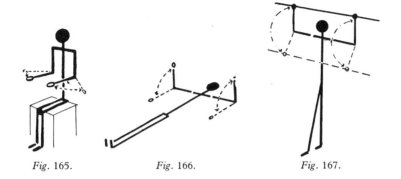

Fig. 165.          Fig. 166.                    Fig. 167.

## 13. MEDIAL ROTATORS OF SHOULDER JOINT

### Strengthening Exercises

*Elementary*

GRADE 1

    1. Forearm reach sitting; single or double Arm turning inwards.

    2. Sitting; Arm turning inwards.

GRADE 2

    1. Heave lying; single or double Arm turning inwards through 90°
(*Fig.* 168).

    2. No progression.

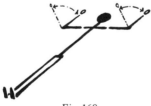

Fig. 168.

GRADE 3

    1. No progression.

    2. Sitting; single or double Hand placing on lumbar spine or slight
distance behind it.


*Intermediate*

GRADE 1

    1. Heave grasp lying (stick crosswise); Arm turning inwards through 90°.

    2. As Exercise 2, in previous grade, but performed in prone lying.

## 14. LATERAL AND MEDIAL ROTATORS OF SHOULDER JOINT

Many of the movements given in the two previous sections may be combined to give wide-range rotation exercises of the shoulder joint. Two examples of mobilizing exercises are given here.

1. Forearm reach sitting; Arm turning outwards and inwards continuously to a given count.

2. Sitting; alternate Hand placing behind the neck and the lumbar spine.

## 15. SHOULDER CIRCUMDUCTORS AND ELEVATORS OF ARM

### Mobilizing Exercises

*Elementary*

GRADE 1

1. Bend sitting; single or double Elbow circling forwards or backwards.
2. Bend sitting; alternate Elbow circling forwards or backwards.

GRADE 2

No progressions.

GRADE 3

1. Sitting or walk-forwards standing; single or double Arm circling forwards or backwards.

1a. Sitting or walk-forwards standing; alternate Arm circling forwards or backwards.

2. Stride standing; single Arm circling in the frontal plane, the circling starting in an outwards or inwards direction.

2a. As Exercise 2, but both arms are moved together and in the same direction.

*Intermediate*

GRADE 1

1. Walk-forwards standing; single or double Arm swinging in a circle: forwards or backwards.

1a. Walk-forwards standing; alternate Arm swinging in a circle: forwards or backwards.

1b. Fallout forwards standing (hand on thigh); single Arm swinging in a circle: forwards or backwards (*Fig.* 169).

2. Stride standing; single Arm swinging in a circle in the frontal plane, the circling starting in an outwards or inwards direction.

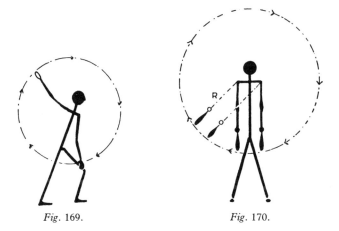

Fig. 169.                              Fig. 170.

2a. As Exercise 2, but the arms are moved together and in the same direction.

GRADE 2

1. Wide grasp walk-forwards standing (stick crosswise in front of body); Arm circling forwards-upwards (Arm bending to bring stick close to chest, stretching forwards-upwards to stretch position, and lowering downwards-forwards to starting position).*

1a–2. No progressions.

2a. Wide grasp stride standing (stick crosswise in front of body); Arm swinging in a circle in the frontal plane, the circling starting to the right or left.*

*Advanced*

GRADE 1

1. Grasp walk-forwards standing (Indian clubs); single or double Arm swinging in a forwards or backwards circle.

1a, b. No progressions.

2. Grasp stride standing (Indian clubs); single Arm swinging in a circle in the frontal plane, the circling starting in an outwards or inwards direction.

2a. As Exercise 2, but the arms are moved together and in the same direction (*Fig.* 170).

GRADE 2

1. Grasp walk-forwards standing (Indian clubs); single Arm swinging in a forwards circle, pausing in the half high reach position to swing the club backwards *behind* the forearm to 1 count.

---

* *See* footnote, p. 120.

1a, b. No progressions.

1c. As Exercise 1, but the arms are moved together.

2. Grasp stride standing (Indian clubs); single Arm swinging in a circle in the frontal plane, pausing in the half high yard position to circle the club backwards *behind* the forearm to 1 count.

2a. As Exercise 2, but the arms are moved together.


## Strengthening Exercises

*See* Exercises in previous section. The movements are performed more slowly than when used as mobility exercises.

# 13. Elbow exercises

**FLEXORS**

**Strengthening Exercises**

*Elementary*

GRADE 1

1. Sitting (forearms and hands resting on table, with elbows flexed and forearms supinated); single Biceps contractions.

GRADE 2

1. No progression.
2. Lying; single or double Elbow bending through 90°.

GRADE 3

1. No progression.
2. Sitting; single or double Elbow bending.

*Intermediate*

GRADE 1

1. No progression.
2. Grasp standing (stick crosswise in front of body); Arm bending.*
3. Reach grasp stoop stride standing (stick crosswise in front of body); Arm bending to bring stick to chest. (*See Fig.* 163, p. 133.)*

GRADE 2

1–3. No progressions.
4. Grasp stride standing (Indian clubs); single Arm swinging across the chest, bending (allowing the upper arm to return to side of trunk), and club circling backwards *behind* the forearm to 3 counts, and stretching downwards.
4a. As previous exercise, but both arms are moved together.
5. Stretch grasp high stoop standing (wall bars); Arm bending. (*See Fig.* 159, p. 129.)

---

* *Stick Exercises*: The types of sticks used for these exercises are broomsticks and ash sticks. Because they are lighter, broomsticks are more useful for early remedial work.

6. Over grasp fall hanging (beam at shoulder height); Arm bending. (*See Fig.* 76, p. 77.)

*Advanced*

GRADE 1

1–4a. No progressions.

5. Angle hanging (wall bars and living support); Arm bending. (*See Fig.* 160, p. 129.)

6. Over grasp fall hanging (beam below shoulder height); Arm bending.

7. Under grasp or over grasp hanging (beam slightly above head height); Arm bending with take-off from floor. (*See Fig.* 157, p. 128, and *Fig.* 171, of Arm bending without take-off.)

GRADE 2

1–5. No progressions.

6. Over grasp horizontal fall hanging (beam and living support); Arm bending. (*See Fig.* 78, p. 78.)

7. Under grasp or over grasp hanging (beam); Arm bending. *Fig.* 171 shows Arm bending from over grasp hanging. (*See also Fig.* 157, p. 128.)

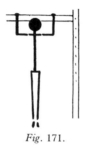

*Fig.* 171.

## EXTENSORS

### Strengthening Exercises

*Elementary*

GRADE 1

1. Sitting; single Triceps contractions.

1a. Lying; single Arm pressing downwards.

GRADE 2

1–1a. No progressions.

2. Bend lying; single or double Arm stretching forwards.

GRADE 3

1–1a. No progressions.

2. Bend sitting; single or double Arm stretching sideways-upwards.

*Intermediate*

GRADE 1

1–1a. No progressions.

2. Bend grasp sitting (stick crosswise); Arm stretching sideways-upwards.*

GRADE 2

1–2. No progressions.

3. Grasp stride standing (Indian clubs); single Arm swinging in a circle in the frontal plane (the circling starting in an outwards or inwards direction), pausing in the half stretch position to (*a*) bend the arm, so that the hand is brought behind the head, and (*b*) circle the club backwards *behind* the forearm to 3 counts.

4. Inclined prone falling (wall bars: hands between shoulder and hip height); Arm bending. (*See Fig.* 162, p. 131.)

*Advanced*

GRADE 1

1–3. No progressions.

4. Inclined prone falling (beam below hip height: hands supported); Arm bending. (*See Fig.* 62, p. 71.)

GRADE 2

1–3. No progressions.

4. Horizontal prone falling; Arm bending. (*See Fig.* 66, p. 72.)

## FLEXORS AND EXTENSORS

### Strengthening Exercises

*Elementary*

GRADE 1

1. Lying; single or double Elbow bending.

GRADE 2

1. Bend sitting; single or double Arm stretching forwards.
1a. Bend sitting; Arm stretching forwards and sideways.

---

* *See* footnote, p. 139.

*Intermediate*

No progressions.


*Advanced*

GRADE 1

1. Fist bend walk-forwards standing; single Arm punching forwards, and strong return movement.

1a. Fist bend stride standing; single Arm punching sideways, and strong return movement.


## Mobilizing Exercises

*Elementary*

GRADE 2

1. Sitting or walk-forwards standing; alternate Elbow bending and stretching, the extremes of both movements being emphasized.

2. As above, but elbow flexion is combined with supination of forearm, and elbow extension is combined with pronation of forearm.


*Intermediate*

GRADE 1

1. Walk-forwards standing; single Elbow bending and stretching, with gentle rhythmical pressing to 3 counts on reaching the extremes of movement.

2. No progression.

3. Wide grasp stride standing (stick crosswise in front of body); Arm circling forwards-upwards (Arm bending to bring stick to chest, stretching forwards-upwards to stretch position, and lowering downwards-forwards to starting position).*

---

* *See* footnote, p. 139.

# 14. Forearm, wrist and hand exercises

The weight of the moving part in these exercises is relatively small; hence it is impracticable to give lists of progressive exercises as in previous chapters. Specimen exercises for the individual muscle groups are listed.

## 1. *FOREARM EXERCISES*

### PRONATORS

#### Strengthening Exercises

*Elementary*

1. Sitting (elbows flexed to 90°, with palms together and fingers pointing forwards-downwards); single or double Forearm pronation.

*Intermediate*

2. Half forearm reach grasp standing (stick vertical with distal end pointing downwards: hand grasps shaft some distance from proximal end); single Forearm turning inwards until stick is in horizontal position with distal end pointing outwards. *Fig.* 172 shows the exercise taken from walk forwards standing.*

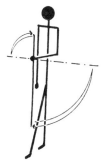

*Fig.* 172.

---

* *Stick Exercises*: The types of sticks used for these exercises are broomsticks and ash sticks. Because they are lighter, broomsticks are more useful for early remedial work.

3. Starting position as above, but distal end of stick points upwards; single Forearm turning outwards until stick is in horizontal position with distal end pointing outwards.*

*Advanced*

4. Stick exercises as above, but hand grasps the stick close to the proximal end.*

## SUPINATORS

### Strengthening Exercises

*Elementary*

1. Forearm reach sitting (palms downwards, lax wrists and fingers); single or double Forearm supination, so that the fingers point upwards. *Fig.* 165, p. 135, shows Forearm reach position.

*Intermediate*

2. Half forearm reach grasp standing (stick vertical with distal end pointing downwards: hand grasps shaft some distance from proximal end); single Forearm turning outwards until stick is in horizontal position with distal end pointing inwards. *Fig.* 173 shows the exercise taken from walk-forwards standing.*

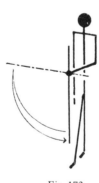

*Fig.* 173

2a. Starting position as above, but distal end of stick points upwards; single Forearm turning inwards until stick is in horizontal position with distal end pointing inwards.*

---

* *See* footnote, p. 143.

*Advanced*

3. Stick exercises as above, but the hand grasps the stick close to the proximal end.*

## PRONATORS AND SUPINATORS
### Strengthening Exercises
*Elementary*

1. Forearm reach sitting (lax fingers); single or double Forearm turning. *Fig.* 165, p. 135, shows Forearm reach position.

*Intermediate*

2. 'Screwing' inwards and outwards movements with a stick against self-resistance (*Fig.* 174).*

3. Half forearm reach grasp standing (palm downwards, and stick horizontal, with distal end pointing outwards: hand grasps shaft some distance from proximal end); single Forearm turning outwards until stick is in horizontal position with distal end pointing inwards (*Fig.* 175).*

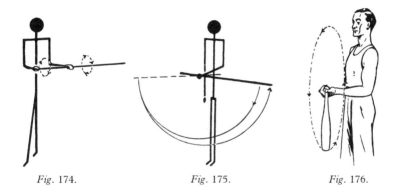

Fig. 174.                    Fig. 175.                    Fig. 176.

3a. Starting position as above, but palm faces upwards; single Forearm turning inwards until stick is in horizontal position with distal end pointing inwards.*

*Advanced*

4. Stick exercises as above. In the 'screwing' movements the self-resistance is increased, and in the Forearm turning exercises the hand grasps the stick close to the proximal end.

* *See* footnote, p. 143.

5. Grasp stride standing (Indian clubs); single Elbow bending to 90°, and club swinging in a circle in an outwards or inwards direction. *Fig.* 176 shows a swinging which starts in an outwards direction.

5a. As Exercise 5, but both arms are used at the same time.

6. Grasp walk-forwards standing (Indian clubs); single Arm swinging forwards-upwards, and club circling (*a*) backwards *behind* the forearm to 2 counts, and (*b*) backwards *in front* of the forearm to 2 counts.

6a. As Exercise 6, but both arms are moved at the same time.

## Mobilizing Exercises

*Elementary*

1. Forearm reach sitting (lax fingers); single, double, or alternate Forearm turning inwards and outwards.

*Intermediate*

2. Forearm reach sitting (lax fingers); single or double Forearm turning inwards and outwards with rhythmical pressing to a given count.

3. Forearm reach sitting (lax wrists and fingers); alternate Forearm turning inwards and outwards with a shaking motion.

4. Sitting or walk-forwards standing; alternate Elbow bending (with Forearm supination) and stretching (with Forearm pronation).

5. Half Forearm reach grasp standing (stick in vertical position, and grasped at centre of shaft); single Forearm turning inwards and outwards with a swinging motion.

6. 'Screwing' inwards and outwards movements with a stick. (*See Fig.* 174, p. 145.)

*Advanced*

*See* Club Exercises in previous section.

## 2. WRIST EXERCISES

The muscles of the wrist are exercised synergically when the fingers are used, e.g. in gripping, the wrist extensors act synergically. Exercises and simple occupations for the fingers should always be used in association with specific wrist exercises.

## WRIST FLEXORS
### Strengthening Exercises
*Elementary*

1. Forearm reach sitting (palms upwards, lax fingers); single or double Wrist flexion (*Fig.* 177).
2. As above, but with Finger flexion.

*Intermediate*

3. Half grasp standing (palm forwards, and stick held obliquely forwards with distal end resting on floor: hand grasps shaft some distance from proximal end); single Wrist bending (*Fig.* 178).*

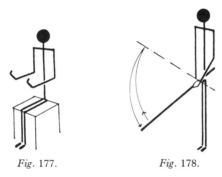

Fig. 177.                    Fig. 178.

4. Forearm reach grasp standing (palms upwards: stick crosswise); Wrist flexion. *Fig.* 165, p. 135, shows Forearm reach position.*

*Advanced*

5. As Exercise 3, but the hand grasps the stick close to the proximal end.*

## WRIST EXTENSORS
### Strengthening Exercises
*Elementary*

1. Forearm reach sitting (palms downwards, lax fingers and wrists); single or double Wrist extension. *Fig.* 165, p. 135, shows Forearm reach position.
2. As Exercise 1, but with Finger extension.

---

* *See* footnote, p. 143.

*Intermediate*

3. Half grasp standing (palm backwards, and stick held obliquely forward with distal end resting on floor: hand grasps shaft some distance from proximal end); single Wrist extension (*Fig.* 179).*

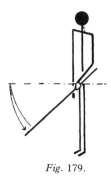

*Fig.* 179.

4. Forearm reach grasp standing (palms downwards: stick crosswise); Wrist extension. *Fig.* 165, p. 135, shows Forearm reach position.*

*Advanced*

5. As Exercise 3, but the hand grasps the stick close to the proximal end.*

## WRIST FLEXORS AND EXTENSORS
### Strengthening Exercises
*Elementary*

1. Sitting (forearms and hands supported on table, palms facing inwards and fingers lax); single or double Wrist flexion and extension, and return to starting position.
2. As above, but performed from Forearm reach sitting.

### Mobilizing Exercises
*Elementary*

1. Forearm reach sitting (lax fingers); alternate Wrist flexion and extension. (*See Fig.* 180, which shows a modified position of forearms.

---

* *See* footnote, p. 143.

*Intermediate*

2. Forearm reach sitting (lax fingers); single Wrist flexion and extension, with gentle rhythmical pressing to a given count on reaching the extremes of movement.

3. Forearm reach sitting or standing (palms downwards, lax fingers and wrists); alternate Wrist flexion and extension with a shaking motion (*Fig.* 180).

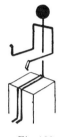

*Fig.* 180.

4. Standing or sitting (fingers interlocked, with elbows flexed and arms to sides); alternate Wrist flexion and extension.

## WRIST ABDUCTORS

### Strengthening Exercises

*Elementary*

1. Sitting (hands and forearms supported on table, palms facing inwards and fingers lax); single or double Wrist abduction.

2. As above, but with fingers straight.

*Intermediate*

3. Half grasp standing (palm inwards, and stick held obliquely forward with distal end resting on floor: hand grasps shaft some distance from proximal end); single Wrist abduction. (*See Fig.* 179, p. 148.)*

*Advanced*

4. As Exercise 3, but the hand grasps the stick close to the proximal end.*

---

* *See* footnote, p. 143.

## WRIST ADDUCTORS
### Strengthening Exercises
*Elementary*

1. Sitting (forearms and hands resting on table, palms facing inwards, fingers lax); single or double Wrist adduction.
2. As above, but the fingers are kept straight.

## WRIST ABDUCTORS AND ADDUCTORS
### Mobilizing Exercises
*Elementary*

1. Sitting (forearms and hands resting on table, palms downwards and fingers lax); alternate Wrist abduction and adduction.
2. As Exercise 1, but the fingers are kept straight.

*Intermediate*

3. As previous exercises, but with gentle rhythmical pressing to a given count on reaching the extremes of movement.

## WRIST CIRCUMDUCTORS
### Mobilizing Exercises
*Elementary*

1. Forearm reach sitting (lax fingers); single or double Wrist circling. *Fig.* 165, p. 135, shows Forearm reach position.

*Advanced*

2. Grasp stride standing (Indian clubs); single Elbow bending to 90°, and club swinging in a circle in an outwards or inwards direction. (*See Fig.* 176, p. 145.)
2a. As above, but both arms are used together.
3. Grasp walk-forwards standing (Indian clubs); single Arm swinging forwards, and club circling (*a*) backwards *behind* the forearm to 2 counts, and (*b*) backwards *in front* of the forearm to 2 counts.
3a. As above, but both arms are moved together.

### Strengthening Exercises
*Advanced*
*See* Club Exercises, above.

## 3. HAND EXERCISES

Simple occupations and everyday activities for the hand should always be used in association with specific exercises for the fingers and thumb.

## EXERCISES TO STRENGTHEN THE GRIP

*Elementary*

1. Forearm reach sitting (lax fingers); strong Finger and Thumb bending, and slow recoil: each hand in turn or both hands together. *Fig.* 165, p. 135, shows Forearm reach position.

2. Sitting; squeezing a sorbo-rubber ball.

3. Sitting (corner of sheet of newspaper held in hand); rolling up paper into a tight ball in the palm of the hand without assistance from the free hand.

4. Sitting (end of unrolled crêpe bandage held in hand); rolling up bandage into a ball in the palm of the hand without assistance from the free hand.

*Intermediate*

5. Standing; stick travelling upwards and downwards, the hands changing places alternately (*Fig.* 181).*

6. As Exercise 5, but the stick is held in one hand, and the grasp is loosened and tightened alternately during the 'travelling'.*

7. Standing; stick throwing from hand to hand (*Fig.* 182).*

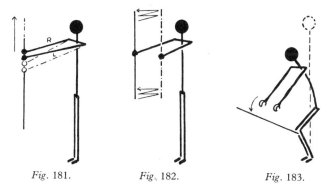

Fig. 181.          Fig. 182.          Fig. 183.

8. Reach grasp standing (stick crosswise); releasing stick and 'dropping' the arms to catch it in the hands again.*

9. Bend grasp standing (stick crosswise); stick throwing upwards and catching.*

10. Reach standing (palms downwards: stick rests crosswise on arms); Arm lowering and stick catching (*Fig.* 183).*

* *See* footnote, p. 143.

11. Inward grasp fall hanging (2 ropes); Arm bending. (*See Fig.* 76, p. 77, where a beam is shown in place of ropes.)

12. Stretch grasp standing (1 or 2 ropes); Arm bending with Ankle stretching to take weight off feet.

*Advanced*

13. Inward grasp horizontal fall hanging (2 ropes and living support); Arm bending. (*See Fig.* 78, p. 78, where a beam is shown in place of ropes.)

14. Over or under grasp hanging (beam); Arm bending. (*See Figs.* 157 and 171, pp. 128 and 140.)

15. Heave grasp walk-forwards standing (rings or ropes); circling and return circling with bent knees, touching the floor with the feet at the end of the forwards circling movement. (*See Fig.* 71, p. 74, which shows a progression on the exercise.)

16. Rope climbing with Leg grasp.

## EXERCISES TO STRENGTHEN THE FINGER AND THUMB EXTENSORS

*Elementary*

1. Sitting (forearms and hands resting on table, palms downwards); Finger and Thumb extension: each hand in turn, or both hands together.

2. Forearm reach sitting (lax fingers); exercise as above.

## EXERCISES TO INCREASE THE RANGE OF FINGER FLEXION OR EXTENSION

*See* Exercises given in two previous groups. Other exercises consist of: (*a*) Finger flexion or extension with rhythmical pressing to a given count, and (*b*) Wide range flexion and extension of the fingers and thumb.

Examples:  (i) *Half forearm reach (lax fingers); Finger flexion with rhyth-mical pressing to 3 counts.* Fig. 165, p. 135, shows Forearm reach position.

(ii) *Forearm reach sitting; Finger and Thumb bending and stretching: each hand in turn, or both hands together.*

## EXERCISES TO STRENGTHEN THE INTRINSIC MUSCLES

*Elementary*

1. Sitting (forearms and hands resting on table, palms downwards); single or double Hand shortening (flexion of the metacarpophalangeal joints with the interphalangeal joints kept extended).

2. Starting position as above; Finger or Thumb parting, closing and relaxation: each hand in turn, or both hands together.

3. Sitting (palms of hands together in front of chest, with fingers pointing upwards and thumbs extended); Hand shortening (pressing finger tips together with flexion of the metacarpophalangeal joints—the interphalangeal joints being kept extended—and opposition of carpo-metacarpal joints).


## EXERCISES TO STRENGTHEN THE THENAR AND HYPOTHENAR MUSCLES

*See* Exercises to Strengthen the Grip, pp. 151–152. Examples of some localized exercises of an elementary grade are given below.

1. Forearm reach sitting (lax fingers); 'making O's' (touching the tip of each finger in turn with the tip of the thumb): each hand in turn, or both hands together. *Fig.* 165, p. 135, shows Forearm reach position.

2. Forearm reach sitting (palms upwards, lax fingers); Palm hollowing (opposition of Thumb and 5th Finger): each hand in turn, or both hands together.

3. Forearm reach sitting; single or double Thumb circling slowly.

4. Forearm reach sitting (palms upwards); single or double Thumb abduction and adduction.

# 15. Hip exercises

Certain hip exercises in which the lower limbs are moved on the trunk are associated with movements of the pelvis and lumbar spine. These associated hip and trunk movements are described in the chapter on trunk exercises (pp. 69–108).

When leg exercises are used to activate the hip muscles the lower limbs ought not to be moved together as, for example, in *Leg raising* from lying. 'Double leg' exercises have a greater specific effect on the spinal muscles.


## HIP FLEXORS
### Strengthening Exercises
(*See also* Exercises for the Flexors of the Spine, pp. 69–76.)


*Elementary*

GRADE 1
    1. Lying; single Knee raising. (*See* p. 69.)

GRADE 2
    1. Lying; single high Knee raising. (*See Fig.* 59, p. 70.)


*Intermediate*

GRADE 1
    1. Low grasp back towards standing (wall bars); single high Knee raising (*Fig.* 184).
    2. Lying; single Leg raising to 45°.
    2a. Lying; single Leg raising.
    3. Lying; single high Knee raising, Leg stretching forwards to 45°, and lowering.

GRADE 2
    1. No progression.

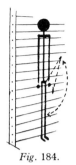

*Fig.* 184.

2. Low grasp back towards standing (wall bars); single Leg raising to 45°.
2a. As above, but single Leg raising.

## Mobilizing Exercises

*Elementary*
  1. Lying; alternate Knee raising.
  2. Lying; alternate high Knee raising.

*Intermediate*
  1. No progression.
  2. Lying; cycling.

## HIP EXTENSORS

### Strengthening Exercises

(*See also* Exercises for the Extensors of the Spine, pp. 76–85. Hopping and Skipping Exercises may also be included.)

*Elementary*

GRADE 1
  1. Lying or prone lying; single or double Gluteal contractions.
  2. Lying; single Leg down pressing.

GRADE 2
  1–2. No progressions.
  3. Reach grasp standing (wall bars or chair back); single Leg raising backwards.

*Intermediate*

GRADE 1

1–2. No progressions.

3. Forehead rest prone lying; single Leg raising backwards.

4. Low reach grasp standing (wall bars); Heel raising and Knee bending. (*See Fig.* 194, p. 165.)

5. Low reach grasp high standing (wall bars and balance bench); stepping down backwards, sound Leg leading (1–2), and stepping up forwards, sound Leg leading (3–4). (*See Fig.* 195, p. 165.)

6. Climbing the wall bars, 1–2 bars at a step.

GRADE 2

1–2. No progressions.

3. Prone kneeling; single Leg stretching and raising backwards. (*See* leg movement of *Fig.* 98*b*, p. 86.)

4. Half wing half low yard grasp standing (wall bars); Heel raising and Knee bending (*Fig.* 185).

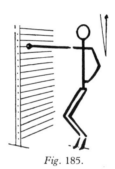

*Fig.* 185.

5. Reach grasp standing (wall bars and balance bench); stepping up forwards, affected Leg leading (1–2), and stepping down backwards, affected Leg leading (3–4).

6. Climbing the wall bars, 2–3 bars at a step.

7. Low reach grasp instep support standing (wall bars and stool); single Heel raising and Knee bending. (*See Fig.* 188, p. 157), which shows a progression on the exercise.)

8. Low reach grasp standing (wall bars); Heel raising and Knee full bending.

*Advanced*

GRADE 1

1–3. No progressions.

4. Wing standing; Heel raising and Knee bending.

5. Toward standing (balance bench or stool); stepping up forwards, affected Leg leading (1–2), and stepping down backwards, affected Leg leading (3–4).

6. No progression.

7. Half wing half low yard grasp instep support standing (wall bars and stool); single Heel raising and Knee bending. (*See Fig.* 185 for position of arms, and *Fig.* 188 for movement.)

8. Half wing half low yard grasp standing (wall bars); Heel raising and Knee full bending.

9. Low reach grasp high half standing (wall bars and plinth); single Knee full bending (*Fig.* 186).

GRADE 2

1–3. No progressions.

4. Neck rest standing; Heel raising and Knee bending.

5. Back toward standing (balance bench or stool); stepping up backwards, affected Leg leading (1–2), and stepping down forwards, affected Leg leading (3–4) (*Fig.* 187).

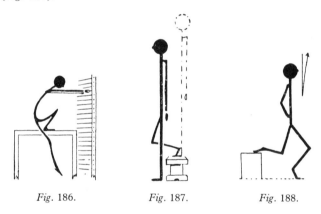

Fig. 186.          Fig. 187.          Fig. 188.

6. No progression.

7. Wing instep support standing (stool); single Heel raising and Knee bending (*Fig.* 188).

8. Wing standing; Heel raising and Knee full bending.

9. Half low yard grasp high half standing (wall bars and plinth); single Knee full bending.

GRADE 3

1–3. No progressions.

4. Stretch standing; Heel raising and Knee bending

5–6. No progressions.

7. Stretch instep support (stool); single Heel raising and Knee bending.

8. Neck rest standing; Heel raising and Knee full bending.

9. Lax reach high half standing (plinth or high bench); single Knee full bending. (*See Fig.* 200, p. 167.)

## Mobilizing Exercises

*Intermediate*

GRADE 1

1. Forehead rest prone lying; single Leg raising backwards with rhythmical pressing to 3 counts.

2. Bend grasp high standing (wall bars); Knee full bending and stretching with Hand travelling down and up the bars. (*See Fig.* 206, p. 169.)

GRADE 2

1. Prone kneeling; single Leg stretching and raising backwards, with rhythmical pressing to 3 counts. (*See* leg movement of *Fig.* 98*b*, p. 86.)

2. No progression.

## HIP FLEXORS AND EXTENSORS

### Strengthening Exercises

(*See also* Exercises for the Flexors and Extensors of the Spine, pp. 85–91.)

*Elementary*

GRADE 1

1. Half crook side-lying; single slight Leg raising sideways, and carrying forwards and backwards, and return to starting position.

GRADE 2

1. Lying; single high Knee raising, and return to starting position, followed by Leg downpressing.

*Intermediate*

GRADE 1

1. Reach grasp standing (wall bars); single high Knee raising, Leg stretching and raising backwards, and return to starting position.

2. Prone kneeling; single high Knee raising, Leg stretching and raising backwards, and return to starting position.

## Mobilizing Exercises

*Elementary*

1. Half crook side-lying; single slight Leg raising sideways, and carrying forwards and backwards to a given count (*Fig.* 189).
2. As above, but the Leg is swung forwards and backwards.

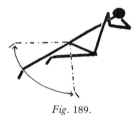

*Fig.* 189.

*Intermediate*

1. No progression.
2. Reach grasp high half standing (beam and block); single Leg swinging forwards and backwards.

## HIP ABDUCTORS

### Strengthening Exercises

(*See also* Exercises for the Lateral Flexors of the Spine, pp. 92–99.)

*Elementary*

GRADE 1

1. Reach grasp standing (wall bars); single Leg raising sideways.
2. Reach grasp standing (wall bars); single slight Knee raising (activates hip abductors of standing leg).
3. Hanging (wall bars or beam); Leg parting.

GRADE 2

1. Standing; single Leg raising sideways.
2. Standing; single Knee raising.
3. Half crook side-lying; single Leg raising sideways.

## HIP ADDUCTORS

### Strengthening Exercises

(*See also* Exercises for the Lateral Flexors of the Spine, pp. 92–99.)

*Elementary*

GRADE 1
  1. Close lying; pressing Knees together.
  2. Crook lying; Knee parting and closing to press the knees together.

GRADE 2
  1. No progression.
  2. Yard (palms on floor) vertical leg lift lying; Leg parting (*Fig.* 190).

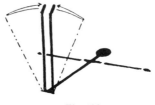

*Fig.* 190.

  2a. Reverse hanging (wall bars); Leg parting. *Fig.* 123, p. 99, shows the reverse hanging position.
  3. Hanging (wall bars or beam); Leg crossing.
  4. Reach grasp high half standing (wall bars and block); single Leg crossing.

## HIP ABDUCTORS AND ADDUCTORS
### Strengthening Exercises
(*See also* Exercises for the Lateral Flexors of the Spine, pp. 92–99.)

*Elementary*

GRADE 1
  1. Lying; single slight Leg raising, and carrying sideways and across the other leg, and return to starting position.
  2. Lying; Leg parting and crossing, and return to starting position.

GRADE 2
  1. Reach grasp standing (wall bars); single Leg raising sideways, lowering and crossing the standing leg, and return to starting position.
  2. Hanging (wall bars or beam); Leg parting and crossing, and return to starting position.

## Mobilizing Exercises

*Elementary*

GRADE 1

1. Lying; single slight Leg raising, and carrying sideways and across the other leg to a given count.

GRADE 2

1. As above, but the Leg is swung from side to side.

*Intermediate*

GRADE 1

1. Reach grasp high half standing (beam and block); single Leg swinging from side to side.

# LATERAL ROTATORS OF HIP

## Strengthening Exercises

*Elementary*

GRADE 1

1. Half crook side-lying; single Leg turning outwards.
2. Crook side-lying; single Knee raising sideways, with feet kept together.

GRADE 2

1–2. No progressions.

3. High sitting (plinth); single Thigh turning outwards, so that foot crosses other leg.

3a. As above, but both Thighs are turned outwards (*Fig.* 191).

4. Prone lying (knees flexed to 90°); allowing Thighs to turn inwards, so that feet are parted (*Fig.* 192).

5. Reach grasp standing (wall bars); Hip turning outwards, feet remaining in starting position.

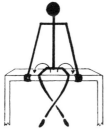

*Fig.* 191.

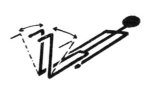

*Fig.* 192.

## MEDIAL ROTATORS OF HIP

### Strengthening Exercises

*Elementary*

GRADE 1

1. Lying (lax legs); Leg turning inwards.
2. Crook lying; Knee parting.

GRADE 2

1-2. No progressions.

3. High sitting (plinth); single Thigh turning inwards, so that lower leg moves outwards.

3a. As above, but both Thighs are turned inwards.

4. Stride prone lying (knees flexed to 90°); allowing Thighs to turn outwards, so that ankles cross each other (*Fig.* 193).

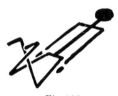

*Fig.* 193.

## LATERAL AND MEDIAL ROTATORS OF HIP

### Strengthening Exercises

(*See also* Exercises for the Rotators of the Spine, pp. 99–103.)

*Elementary*

GRADE 1

1. Reach grasp half standing (wall bars); single Leg turning inwards and outwards, and return to starting position.

2. Stride lying; single or double Leg turning inwards and outwards, and return to starting position.

GRADE 2

1-2. No progressions.

3. High sitting (plinth); single or double Thigh turning inwards and outwards to the full extent, and return to starting position.

4. Prone lying; exercise as above.

5. Half crook lying; single Knee lowering sideways, raising to cross other leg, and return to starting position.

**Mobilizing Exercises**

As strengthening exercises, above, but the movements are performed in a continuous manner, e.g. *Stride lying; single Leg turning inwards and outwards continuously to a given count.* (*See also* Exercises for the Rotators of the Spine, pp. 99–103.)

## CIRCUMDUCTORS OF HIP

**Mobilizing Exercises**

*Elementary*

1. Reach grasp high half standing (beam and block); single Leg circling or swinging in a circle.
2. Lying; single Leg circling.
3. Half crook side-lying; single Leg circling.

**Strengthening Exercises**

*See* Exercises in previous section. The movements are performed more slowly than when used as mobility exercises. *See also* Exercises for the Circumductors of the Spine, pp. 107–108.)

# 16. Knee exercises

**KNEE FLEXORS**

**Strengthening Exercises**

(*See also* single Leg raising backwards exercises, pp. 155–156.)

*Elementary*

GRADE 1
1. Crook lying or sitting; single or double Hamstring contractions.

GRADE 2
1. No progression.
2. Forehead rest prone lying; single or double Knee bending to 90°.

GRADE 3
1. No progression.
2. High sitting (table or bench); single or double Knee bending.
3. Reach grasp standing (wall bars); single Knee bending backwards.

**KNEE EXTENSORS**

**Strengthening Exercises**

(Hopping and Skipping Exercises may also be included.)

*Elementary*

GRADE 1
1. Long sitting (trunk inclined backwards with hand support) or half lying; single or double Quadriceps contractions.
2. As Exercise 1, with Ankle or Foot movements, e.g. single Quadriceps contractions with Ankle bending.

GRADE 2
1. Lying; single Leg raising to 45° with Knee firmly braced.
1a. As above, but with Ankle bending.

2. Lying; single Leg raising with Knee firmly braced.

2a. As above, but with Ankle bending.

3. High sitting (plinth); single or double Knee stretching.

3a. As above, but with Ankle bending.

*Intermediate*

GRADE 1

1. Lying; single high Knee raising, Leg stretching forwards to 45°, and slow lowering.

1a–2a. No progressions.

3. Low reach grasp standing (wall bars); Heel raising and Knee bending (*Fig.* 194).

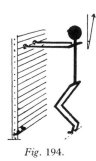 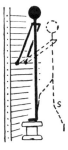 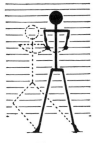

Fig. 194.                    Fig. 195.                    Fig. 196.

4. Low reach grasp high standing (wall bars and balance bench); stepping down backwards, sound Leg leading (1–2), and stepping up forwards, sound Leg leading (3–4) (*Fig.* 195).

5. Climbing the wall bars, 1–2 bars at a step.

GRADE 2

1–2a. No progressions.

3. Half wing half low yard grasp standing (wall bars); Heel raising and Knee bending.

4. Reach grasp standing (wall bars and balance bench); stepping up forwards, affected Leg leading (1–2), and stepping down backwards, affected Leg leading (3–4).

5. Climbing the wall bars, 2–3 bars at a time.

6. Low reach grasp standing (wall bars); Heel raising and Knee full bending.

7. Low reach grasp stride standing (wall bars); Heel raising and single Knee bending (*Fig.* 196).

8. Low reach grasp instep support standing (wall bars and stool); single Heel raising and Knee bending.

9. Short fallout forwards standing; vigorous thrusting backwards (*Fig.* 197).

*Advanced*

GRADE 1

1–2a. No progressions.

3. Wing standing; Heel raising and Knee bending.

4. Towards standing (balance bench or stool); stepping up forwards, affected Leg leading (1–2), and stepping down backwards, affected Leg leading (3–4).

5. No progression.

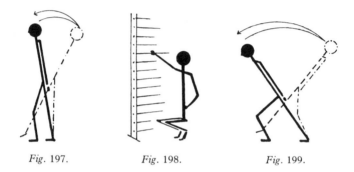

*Fig.* 197.               *Fig.* 198.               *Fig.* 199.

6. Half wing half low yard grasp-standing (wall bars); Heel raising and Knee full bending. (*Fig.* 198)

7. Half wing half low yard grasp stride-standing (wall bars); Heel raising and single Knee bending.

8. Half wing half low yard grasp instep support standing (wall bars and stool); single Heel raising and Knee bending.

8a. Low reach grasp high half standing (wall bars and plinth); single Knee full bending. (*See Fig.* 186, p. 157.)

9. Fallout forwards standing; vigorous thrusting backwards (*Fig.* 199).

GRADE 2

1–2a. No progressions.

3. Neck rest standing; Heel raising and Knee bending.

4. Back towards standing (balance bench or stool); stepping up backwards, affected Leg leading (1–2), and stepping down forwards, affected Leg leading (3–4). (*See Fig.* 187, p. 157.)

5. No progression.

6. Wing standing; Heel raising and Knee full bending.

7. Wing stride-standing; Heel raising and single Knee bending.

8. Wing instep support standing (stool); single Heel raising and Knee bending. (*See Fig.* 188, p. 157.)

8a. Half low yard grasp high half standing (wall bars and plinth); single Knee full bending.

9. No progression.

GRADE 3

1–2a. No progressions.

3. Stretch standing; Heel raising and Knee bending.

4–5. No progressions.

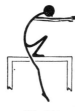

*Fig.* 200.

6. Neck rest standing; Heel raising and Knee full bending.

7. Neck rest stride standing; Heel raising and single Knee bending.

8. Neck rest instep support standing (stool); single Heel raising and Knee bending. *See Fig.* 188, p. 157, which shows the arms in wing position.

8a. Lax reach high half standing (plinth); single Knee full bending (*Fig.* 200).

9. No progression.

## KNEE ROTATORS

Specific exercises for the knee rotators are not given here, because rotation of the knee is associated with flexion and extension movements. *See* Exercises for the Knee Flexors, p. 164, and Exercises for the Knee Extensors, pp. 164–167.

## KNEE FLEXORS AND EXTENSORS

### Strengthening Exercises

Knee flexion and extension movements may be combined in half crook side-lying and high sitting, e.g. *High sitting (table or bench); single or double Knee bending, stretching, and return to starting position.* (*Fig.* 201.)

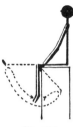

*Fig.* 201.

## EXERCISES TO RESTORE THE RANGE OF KNEE FLEXION

### a. For use when the range of Knee flexion is less than 45°

1. Lying; affected Knee raising with heel in contact with supporting surface.

2. Half crook side-lying; affected Knee bending and stretching continuously to a given count.

3. Prone lying; alternate Knee bending.

4. Prone lying; affected Knee bending with rhythmical pressing to a given count.

5. High sitting (plinth: heels resting on stool, with knees flexed); alternate Knee stretching.

### b. For use when the range of Knee flexion is between 45° and 90°

1. Lying; affected Knee raising with heel in contact with supporting surface.

2. Half crook side-lying; affected Knee bending and stretching continuously to a given count.

3. Prone lying; alternate Knee bending.

4. Prone lying; affected Knee bending with rhythmical pressing to a given count.

5. High sitting (table or bench); alternate Knee stretching.

6. As above; alternate lower Leg swinging with Ankle bending and stretching (*Fig.* 202).

7. High sitting (table or bench); affected Knee attempted bending beyond stiff zone, and slow recoil.

8. Prone kneeling (knee position modified if necessary); Trunk moving backwards and forwards. (*See Fig.* 205, p. 169.)

8a. As Exercise 8, but with rhythmical pressing to a given count at end of backwards movement.

9. Short walk-forwards standing (hands on forward knee); small range bending and stretching of forward knee (*Fig.* 203).

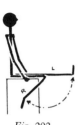

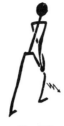

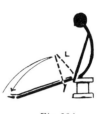

Fig. 202. Fig. 203. Fig. 204.

10. Low grasp inclined long sitting (balance bench); single high Knee raising, attempting to touch front edge of bench with heel (*Fig.* 204).

11. Bend grasp high standing (wall bars); Knee bending and stretching with Hand travelling down and up the bars. *Fig.* 206, shows Hand travelling over two bars only.

### c. For use when the range of Knee flexion is over 90°

1–2. Omitted.

3. Prone lying; alternate Knee bending.

4. Prone lying; affected Knee bending with rhythmical pressing to a given count.

5. Omitted.

6. High sitting (table or bench); alternate lower Leg swinging forwards and backwards with Ankle bending and stretching (*Fig.* 202).

7. High sitting (table or bench); affected Knee bending as far as possible, and slow recoil.

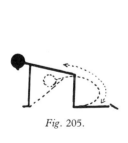

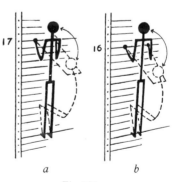

Fig. 205. a b

Fig. 206.

8. Prone kneeling; Trunk moving backwards and forwards (*Fig.* 205).

8a. As above, but with rhythmical pressing to a given count at end of the backwards movement.

9. Fallout forwards standing (hands on forward knee); small range bending and stretching of forward knee. (*See Fig.* 203, p. 169.)

10. As Exercise 10, previous section.

11. Bend grasp high standing (wall bars); Knee bending and stretching with Hand travelling down and up the bars. *Fig.* 206 shows Hand travelling over two bars only.

12. Lax stoop half kneeling (hands on floor); small range bending and stretching of forward knee (*Fig.* 207).

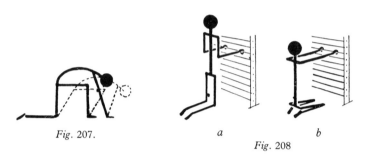

Fig. 207.                         a                         b

Fig. 208

13. Forearm reach grasp kneeling (wall bars); attempting to assume kneel sitting (*Fig.* 208).

# 17. Ankle and foot exercises

## 1. ANKLE EXERCISES

### DORSIFLEXORS

#### Strengthening Exercises

(Balance Exercises may also be included.)

*Elementary*

GRADE 1

1. Half lying or long sitting with trunk inclined backwards and hand support (heels free); single or double Ankle bending with slight Knee raising.
2. As above, but without Knee raising.

GRADE 2

1. High sitting (plinth); single or double Ankle bending.
2. No progression.
3. Sitting; single or double Forefoot raising.

*Intermediate*

GRADE 1

1. No progression.
2. Reach grasp standing (wall bars); Forefoot raising.
3. No progression.

### PLANTAR-FLEXORS

#### Strengthening Exercises

(*See also* Exercises for the Knee Extensors, pp. 164–167. Hopping, Skipping, and Balance Exercises may also be included.)

*Elementary*

GRADE 1

1. Long sitting (trunk inclined backwards with hand support) or half lying; single or double Ankle stretching.

GRADE 2
1. Prone lying (plinth: feet free); as previous exercise.

GRADE 3
1. Sitting; single or double Heel raising.


*Intermediate*

GRADE 1
1. Reach grasp standing (wall bars); Heel raising.

GRADE 2
1. Half yard grasp standing (wall bars); Heel raising.
2. Reach grasp instep support standing (wall bars and stool); single Heel raising. (*See Fig.* 209, which shows a progression on this exercise.)


*Advanced*

GRADE 1
1. Wing standing; Heel raising.
1a. Standing; Heel raising with Arm swinging forwards and forwards-upwards.
2. Half yard grasp instep support standing (wall bars and stool); single Heel raising.
3. Walking on the toes with 'springing' steps.

GRADE 2
1. Neck rest standing; Heel raising.
1a. No progression.
2. Wing instep support standing (stool); single Heel raising (*Fig.* 209).

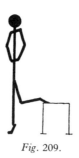

*Fig.* 209.

2a. Lax yard half standing; single Heel raising.
3. Running on the toes.

## DORSIFLEXORS AND PLANTAR-FLEXORS

### Strengthening Exercises

(Balance Exercises may also be included.)

Many of the movements given in the two previous sections may be combined, e.g. *High sitting (plinth); Ankle bending, stretching, and return to starting position.*

### Mobilizing Exercises

*Elementary*

1. Half lying or long sitting with trunk inclined backwards and hand support (heels free); alternate Ankle bending and stretching.

2. High sitting (plinth); as above.

3. Sitting (one ankle crossed over opposite knee); single Ankle bending and stretching continuously to a given count.

4. Sitting; alternate Forefoot and Heel raising (*Fig.* 210).

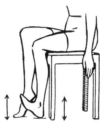

*Fig.* 210.

## 2. FOOT EXERCISES

## INVERTORS

### Strengthening Exercises

(Balance exercises may also be included.)

*Elementary*

GRADE 1

1. Half lying or long sitting with trunk inclined backwards and hand support (heels free); single or double Foot turning inwards.

1a. As Exercise 1, with Toe flexion.

GRADE 2

1. High sitting (plinth); single or double Foot turning inwards.

1a. As Exercise 1, with Toe flexion.

2. Sitting (one ankle crossed over opposite knee); single Foot turning inwards.

3. Sitting; single or double inner Border raising.

4. Sitting; attempting to accentuate medial longitudinal arches.

*Intermediate*

GRADE 1

1–2. No progressions.

3. Reach grasp standing (wall bars) or standing; inner Border raising.

4. Starting position as Exercise 3; attempting to accentuate medial longitudinal arches.

## EVERTORS
### Strengthening Exercises
(Balance exercises may also be included.)

*Elementary*

GRADE 1

1. Half lying or long sitting with trunk inclined backwards and hand support (heels free); single or double Foot turning outwards.

GRADE 2

1. High sitting (plinth); single or double Foot turning outwards.

2. Sitting (one ankle crossed over opposite knee); single Foot turning outwards.

3. Short stride sitting; single or double outer Border raising.

*Intermediate*

GRADE 1

1–2. No progressions.

3. Reach grasp short stride standing (walls bars) or standing; outer Border raising.

## INVERTORS AND EVERTORS
### Strengthening Exercises
(Balance Exercises may also be included.)

Certain of the movements given in the two previous sections may be combined, e.g. *High sitting (plinth); Foot turning inwards and outwards, and return to starting position.*

## Mobilizing Exercises

*Elementary*

1. Half lying or long sitting with trunk inclined backwards and hand support (heels free); alternate Foot turning inwards and outwards continuously to a given count.

2. High sitting (plinth); as above.

3. Sitting (one ankle crossed over opposite knee); single Foot turning inwards and outwards continuously to a given count.

4. Short stride sitting; inner and outer Border raising continuously to a given count.


# CIRCUMDUCTORS

## Mobilizing Exercises

*Elementary*

1. Half lying or long sitting with trunk inclined backwards and hand support (heels free); single or double Foot circling.

2. High sitting (plinth); as above.

3. Sitting (one ankle crossed over opposite knee); single Foot circling.

*N.B.* Emphasis may be placed on a particular part of the circling, e.g. Circling with emphasis on inversion.


## Strengthening Exercises

The movements given in the previous section may also be used as strengthening exercises; they are then performed more slowly.


# INTRINSIC MUSCLES

## Strengthening Exercises

*Elementary*

1. Sitting; single or double Foot shortening (flexion of the metatarsophalangeal joints, with extension of the interphalangeal joints) (*Fig.* 211).

1a. Half lying (feet supported by footboard, with ankles dorsiflexed); single or double Foot shortening. *See above.* (*Fig.* 212.)

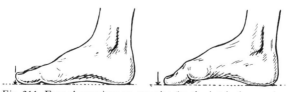

*Fig.* 211. Foot shortening: an exercise for the intrinsic muscles.

2. Half lying or long sitting (trunk inclined backwards with hand support); Toe parting and closing.

2a. Sitting (feet resting on floor or in tray of sand); Toe parting and closing.

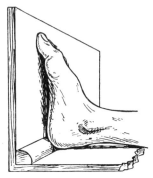

*Fig.* 212. Foot shortening adapted for bed use: the feet are supported by a footboard.

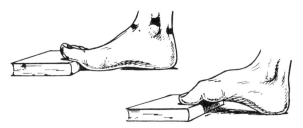

*Fig.* 213. Another exercise for the intrinsic muscles.

3. Sitting (toes resting on book); Toe flexion at the metatarsophalangeal joints, with extension of the interphalangeal joints: each foot in turn, or both together (*Fig.* 213).

4. Sitting (feet resting on book, with all the toes free); Toe flexion at the metatarsophalangeal joints, with extension of the interphalangeal joints: each foot in turn, or both together.

*Intermediate*

1. Standing; single or double Foot shortening. (*See* Exercise 1, Elementary grade).

2. No progression.

3. Standing; practising correct 'push off' movement from toes in walking (interphalangeal joints of toes must be kept extended).

## TOE FLEXORS AND EXTENSORS

The strengthening exercises for the flexors and extensors of the toes consist of strong flexion and extension movements, followed by a slow return to the starting position.

Example: *Half lying or long sitting (trunk inclined backwards with hand support); strong Toe bending, and slow recoil: each foot in turn, or both together.*

The mobilizing exercises consist of flexion and extension movements which are performed in a continuous manner.

Example: *Long sitting (trunk inclined backwards with hand support); Toe bending and stretching continuously to a given count: both feet together.*

# PART 4

# APPLIED EXERCISE THERAPY

# 18. Construction and use of tables of specific exercises

The tables consist of lists of movements which provide exercise for a particular part of the body; they are used in the treatment of localized lesions, such as fractures, chest diseases and postoperative abdominal conditions. A series of graded tables is required to provide smooth, progressive exercise from the early to the late phase of recovery. If a patient's condition remains stationary for a considerable time the exercises are changed or modified to maintain interest.

The patients are treated individually or by group or class methods. In many hospitals and rehabilitation centres men and women are exercised together in the same groups or classes.

*Group and Class Work*

The difference between group and class methods of instruction is not always understood. In group work a small number of patients (6 at the most), with the same or similar types of disability, are treated together. The therapist indicates the exercise to be performed and the patients practise it individually. The therapist goes from patient to patient and gives individual coaching as required.

In class work a number of patients (10–12 at the most), with the same or similar types of disability, exercise in unison under the guidance of the therapist.

*General Exercises*

In rehabilitation centres general exercises and games are used in addition to specific exercises. In hospital rehabilitation departments the limited amount of time available for treatment makes it difficult to organize full-scale general exercise classes. The difficulty can be overcome to some extent by arranging short sessions of general 'warming-up' exercises to music before the specific exercise periods (p. 256).

## THE EXERCISE TABLE

The exercises are selected with regard to the aims of treatment and the phase of recovery reached by the patient. In general, the same type of exercises are used for both men and women. Some of the more strenuous exercises, however, are not suitable for women.

One method of compiling and using a table of specific exercises is given here.

## Compiling the Exercise Table

The aims of treatment are divided into two groups: those of primary importance and those of secondary importance. The exercises which are chosen to achieve the aims are also divided into two groups: Primary and Secondary Exercises. This method has been followed in compiling the lists of progressive exercises for the clinical conditions included in the following chapters.

## Using the Exercise Tables

Primary and secondary exercises are used at each exercise period. The secondary exercises are spaced between the primary exercises, e.g. two or three primary exercises are followed by one or two secondary exercises. In this way there is no danger of the affected part being subjected to too concentrated a period of activity. When the table consists of one group of exercises only this suggestion cannot be followed.

### Avoiding Fatigue

Exercises which activate the same muscle groups should not be given consecutively, because this may produce fatigue. Exercises which use the same muscles in association with other muscles, to produce different movements, may follow each other with little danger of over-fatigue. For example, in strengthening the trunk muscles two exercises which use the abdominal muscles as flexors of the spine should not be given consecutively, but a series of exercises in which the abdominal muscles are used as flexors, rotators and lateral flexors of the spine is permissible. Short rest periods are given whenever they are thought to be necessary.

## 'LITTLE-AND-OFTEN' SELF-PRACTICE

To obtain the maximum benefit from specific exercise therapy the patient should practise two or three of the more important exercises from the exercise table on a 'little-and-often' basis during the day. Unfortunately, this aspect of physical treatment is often overlooked.

The exercises selected for self-practice must be simple, and—if the patient

is confined to bed—capable of being performed with the minimum distur-
bance of the bedclothes. For example, *Quadriceps contractions* and *single
straight Leg raising in small range* are the 'key' exercises prescribed for a
patient resting in bed after meniscectomy.


## LISTS OF SPECIFIC EXERCISES

To aid the therapist in planning exercise tables for certain clinical conditions
some lists of progressive exercises are given in the following chapters.
Introductory notes in each chapter describe the conditions for which the
exercises are suitable and give details of the surgical procedures used.

# 19. Exercise therapy after abdominal surgery

This chapter describes the various forms of exercise therapy which may be used in the postoperative treatment of gastrectomy, cholecystectomy, appendicectomy and inguinal, femoral and umbilical herniae. For convenience of description the exercise procedures which are used to prevent postoperative respiratory and circulatory complications have been grouped together as an introductory section.

Preoperative training of the patient in the exercises and techniques to be used is essential. It is also most important that the therapist explains very simply the reasons for the exercises, without in any way alarming the patient or increasing his apprehension of surgery.

## RESPIRATORY COMPLICATIONS

The main causes of postoperative respiratory complications, such as bronchitis, bronchopneumonia and atelectasis, are: (1) Decreased respiratory movement, particularly limitation of diaphragmatic excursion, and (2) Increased amount of mucous secretions in the respiratory passages as a result of some anaesthetic agent irritation, and inhibition (for a variable period) of the normal ciliary action.

### Decreased Respiratory Movement

This means that parts of the lungs are out of action and not expanding fully, especially at the bases. The principal factors that produce this state are pain and associated reflex spasm of the diaphragm.

The respiratory excursion of the diaphragm is especially limited after operations on the upper abdomen, and this is most evident on the 1st postoperative day. The fall of vital capacity may be as low as 20–25 per cent of normal on the 1st postoperative day. It improves gradually over the next six to ten days.

### Increased Amount of Mucous Secretions

Normally the cough reflex ensures that the patient successfully empties his respiratory passages of secretions. After general anaesthesia, with or without postoperative analgesic drugs, the reflex is very often diminished for as long as twenty-four hours; in addition, the patient is disinclined to cough because of the associated pain in his wound.

*Interaction of these Factors*

Both the decreased respiratory movement and the increased amount of secretions lead to pulmonary congestion and the danger of blockage of a main bronchus, or to multiple patchy collapse by blockage of many small bronchioles. The latter complication is specially likely to proceed to bronchial pneumonia, if inadequately dealt with. Bronchopneumonia, however, may arise independently of collapse, due to infected material (often inhaled from the mouth) gaining a foothold on predisposed ground.

**Alteration of Posture**

After major operations, such as gastrectomy and cholecystectomy, the patient is often encouraged to lie flat on his back, and on the left and right side (*Fig.* 214) during the 1st and 2nd postoperative days. He remains in each position for about 1–2 hours at a time.

This routine alteration of posture assists in the drainage of the lungs and is of great importance in the prevention of pulmonary complications, such as atelectasis. It also helps to 'break' any flatulence which may be present. While in the various positions the patient is encouraged to carry out localized breathing exercises at frequent intervals.

Ballinger and Drapanas (1972) emphasize the value of skilled physiotherapy after surgery. 'In the experience of Bendixen and colleagues, chest physiotherapy before and after operation reduces the incidence of atelectasis or pneumonia from 42 to 12 per cent.'

**Postural Drainage**

Should a collapse of a particular area of the lung develop in spite of all precautions, the patient's posture must be modified to secure adequate drainage of the affected part. For example, if the lateral area of the left lower lobe is affected the patient is placed in the right crook side-lying position (*Fig.* 214), and the foot of the bed is raised 30–60 cm. Routine alteration of posture, as previously described, must still be continued, but the patient spends more time in the specific drainage position.

Postural drainage of this type will be reinforced by the use of shakings and coarse vibrations, encouragement of coughing and expectoration of secretions in lying and crook side-lying (the wound area being supported by the patient's hands or a Cough-Lok), and unilateral breathing exercises, e.g. *Crook side-lying (therapist's hand on side of lower chest); lower lateral Costal*

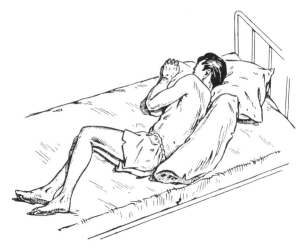

*Fig.* 214. Alteration of posture after major abdominal surgery. The patient is encouraged to lie on his back, and on the left and right side, for about 1–2 hours at a time during the first and second postoperative days. This routine alteration of posture is of great importance in the prevention of pulmonary complications, such as atelectasis.

*breathing,* and *Crook side-lying (therapist's hand on posterior aspect of lower chest); posterior Basal breathing.*

### Postoperative Breathing Exercises

Bilateral breathing exercises are used in the early postoperative days following all forms of abdominal surgery. They are particularly important in the period before the patient is allowed out of bed for the major part of the day.

In addition to being part of regular treatment sessions supervised by the therapist, some of the more important exercises should be carried out by the patient throughout the day on 'little and often' lines.

The starting positions used for the exercises will obviously depend on the patient's condition and the individual preference of the therapist. To avoid repetition *crook lying* and *crook side-lying* are used for the exercises given here.

1. Crook lying and crook side-lying (hand on upper abdomen); Diaphragmatic breathing.* (*See Fig.* 144, p. 110.)
2. Crook lying (hands on sides of lower chest); lower lateral Costal breathing. (*See Fig.* 143, p. 109.)

---

* After gastrectomy and cholecystectomy, where the incisions used involve the upper abdomen (pp. 188–201), diaphragmatic breathing is generally extremely shallow on the 1st postoperative day and may be almost impossible to obtain.

3. Crook lying (hands on sides of upper chest); upper lateral Costal breathing.
4. Crook lying (forearms crossed and fingers resting on chest below clavicles); Apical breathing.
5. Crook lying; general deep breathing.

## CIRCULATORY COMPLICATIONS

'Various factors have been recorded as being responsible for the production of thrombosis and embolism. Three main factors are now recognized as being the possible causes: (a) Increased tendency for the blood to clot, (b) Injury to the intima of the vein at operation, and (c) Slowing of the venous circulation. The last is probably the most important . . . The slowing starts in the second postoperative day and is present until the patient becomes ambulant . . .

'Several competent authorities think that the slowing of the circulation which occurs in the veins of the lower limbs after abdominal surgery is due to interference with the action of the diaphragm. The diaphragm, in addition to fulfilling a respiratory function, also accounts in large measure for the movement of the blood through the veins to the right heart—the pumping action of the diaphragm [by production of intermittent negative pressure in the chest]. As the movements of the diaphragm are much depressed after abdominal surgery, the pumping action is interfered with and consequently slowing of the venous circulation takes place' (Gunn Roberts, 1946).

### Postoperative Leg Exercises

Simple foot, ankle and leg exercises are used during the early postoperative days to accelerate the venous circulation through the lower limbs and pelvis. They are especially important in the period before regular walking is allowed.

In addition to forming part of regular treatment sessions organized by the therapist, some of the more important exercises should be carried out by the patient throughout the day on 'little and often' lines. This is especially important in the period before regular walking is allowed.

Useful exercises, taken in *lying* or *half-lying*, include:
1. Lying; alternate Ankle bending and stretching.
2. Lying; alternate Foot turning inwards and outwards.
3. Lying; single Foot circling.
4. Lying; Toe bending and stretching rhythmically: both feet.
5. Lying; single slight Knee raising and lowering, followed by firm Leg downpressing.
6. Lying; single and double Quadriceps contractions.
7. Lying; combined Quadriceps and Gluteal contractions: alternate legs.

*General Progressions*

8. Sitting over edge of bed; alternate Ankle bending and stretching.
9. Sitting over edge of bed; alternate lower Leg swinging with Ankle bending and stretching.
10. Sitting over edge of bed; single Knee stretching.
11. Sitting (chair); alternate Forefoot raising (1–4), followed by alternate Heel raising (5–8).
12. Sitting (chair); single high Knee raising, lowering and downpressing of Foot on to floor.

---

## 1. GASTRECTOMY*

Partial gastrectomy may be performed in the treatment of peptic ulcer (gastric or duodenal ulcer), and carcinoma of the stomach. Total gastrectomy may be performed for: (1) Carcinoma of the stomach; (2) High gastric ulcer; and (3) Ulcer of the lower end of the oesophagus.

## TYPES OF INCISION

A right upper paramedian incision is commonly used (*Fig.* 215). Sometimes a left upper paramedian incision is used, e.g. in certain cases of gastric ulcer and in carcinoma when wide removal of the stomach is necessary.

The incision is vertical in direction and is situated 1·2–2·5 cm from the midline; it extends approximately from the costal margin to a point one side of the umbilicus (*Fig.* 215).

*Stages of Incision*

1. Incision of skin and subcutaneous tissues, down to the anterior sheath of the rectus muscle.
2. Incision of the anterior sheath of the rectus muscle in the line of the skin incision.
3. Retraction of the rectus muscle laterally, so that no large nerves or vessels are damaged.

---

*a. A gastro-enterostomy (to short-circuit the pyloric part of the stomach and duodenum) is performed by some surgeons for inoperable cases of carcinoma of the pylorus and for pyloric stenosis. A right upper paramedian incision is used. After-treatment by exercise therapy is the same as described for gastrectomy.

*b.* Vagotomy, together with gastro-enterostomy or pyloroplasty, is sometimes performed for cases of duodenal ulcer. A left upper paramedian incision is used; the exercise therapy is as described for gastrectomy.

*c.* Highly selective vagotomy (also known as 'proximal gastric denervation') is now widely used in the treatment of duodenal ulceration.

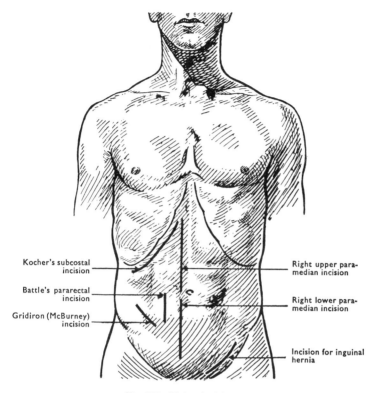

Kocher's subcostal
incision

Battle's pararectal
incision

Gridiron (McBurney)
incision

Right upper para-
median incision

Right lower para-
median incision

Incision for inguinal
hernia

*Fig.* 215. Abdominal incisions.

4. Incision of the posterior rectus sheath and peritoneum in the line of the skin incision.


## EXERCISE AND THE SUTURE LINE

The aponeurosis of the oblique and transverse abdominal muscles form the anterior and posterior sheaths of the rectus muscle. Active trunk rotation will therefore tend to pull more strongly on the suture line than any other form of trunk exercise. When trunk rotation movements are performed they should be of the slow controlled type, and quick jerky movements must be avoided.

Although it is quite possible, and safe, for the average patient to perform simple abdominal exercises of all types on the 1st and 2nd postoperative days, it has been found more convenient in practice to leave these exercises until the 3rd day. Breathing exercises and movements for the lower limbs are essential during the first 2 postoperative days, and usually there is little time for abdominal exercises.

## EXERCISE THERAPY

The lists of progressive exercises given here are intended to be a guide to the after-treatment of partial and total gastrectomy.

## FIRST 2 POSTOPERATIVE DAYS

Usually, intravenous therapy is used on the 1st day, and one of the patient's arms or legs is immobilized for this purpose. A Ryle's tube may be in position for intermittent aspiration of the stomach remnant.

To help prevent pulmonary complications the patient should spend a considerable amount of his time lying flat on his back and on the left and right sides; he stays in each position for about 1–2 hours at a time (p. 185). Should a collapse of a particular area of the lung develop in spite of all precautions, postural drainage will be instituted as outlined on p. 185.

*Sitting out of Bed*

Provided that there are no respiratory complications, sitting out in a chair for about 10–20 minutes is generally allowed on the 1st postoperative day. Supervised walking round the bed is usually allowed on the 2nd day.

*Remedial Aims*

To prevent postoperative respiratory and circulatory complications.

*Exercise Period*

15–20 minutes, two or three times daily. In addition to these treatment sessions the patient will practise some of the exercises on 'little and often' lines.

### Primary Exercises

*Breathing, Ankle/Foot and Leg Exercises* (*see* previous section, pp. 186–188)

It should be noted that diaphragmatic breathing is extremely shallow on the 1st postoperative day and may be almost impossible to obtain (p. 184).

### 3rd and 4th POSTOPERATIVE DAYS

The patient rests in bed between intervals of sitting out in a chair; provided there are no respiratory complications he takes up an ordinary half-lying position. Short periods of walking in the ward are encouraged.

*Remedial Aims*

PRIMARY
1. To prevent postoperative respiratory and circulatory complications.
2. To maintain the abdominal muscles, particularly the oblique and transverse groups.

SECONDARY
1. To maintain the other trunk muscles.
2. To maintain the muscles that support the medial longitudinal arches of the feet.

*Exercise Period*

20 minutes, twice daily. In addition, the patient will practise some of the exercises on 'little and often' lines throughout the day.

## Primary Exercises

*Breathing, Ankle/Foot and Leg Exercises (see* previous section, pp. 186–188
*Trunk Exercises*
1. Crook lying (hand on abdomen); Abdominal contractions.
2. Stride lying; Trunk turning with single Arm carrying across the chest. *See Fig.* 129, p. 101.
3. Lying; Head bending forwards with single high Knee raising. *See Fig.* 50 and *Fig.* 59, p. 62 and 70.

## Secondary Exercises

*Trunk Exercises*
1. Lying; slight Chest raising. (*See Fig.* 80, p. 79, which shows full Chest raising.)
2. Crook lying; Pelvis raising. (*See Fig.* 150, p. 116.)

*Leg Exercises*
1. Half lying; single or double Ankle bending.
2. Half lying; single or double Foot turning inwards.

## 5th TO 10th POSTOPERATIVE DAY

Usually the stitches are removed on the 10th postoperative day, depending on the patient's condition and the surgeon's opinion. (Absorbable cutaneous sutures are sometimes used.) The patient spends an increasing amount of time sitting in a chair. The amount of walking is also increased.

*Remedial Aims*

As for the 3rd and 4th postoperative days. An additional (Primary) aim is to improve posture.

*Exercise Period*

20–30 minutes, once or twice daily.

## 1. PATIENT LYING ON BED

**Primary Exercises**

*Breathing, Ankle/Foot and Leg Exercises*

See pp. 186–188. Because of the patient's increasing mobility the number of exercises used from this section can now be limited to, say, diaphragmatic and lower lateral costal breathing and a general leg movement.

*Trunk Exercises*

1. Stride lying; Trunk turning with Head bending forwards and single Arm carrying across the chest. (*See Fig.* 129, p. 101.)
2. Lying; single high Knee raising, Leg stretching forwards to 45° and slow lowering.
3. Lying (hands grasping edges of mattress); upper Trunk bending forwards with assistance from arms.
4. Heave grasp lying (head posts of bed); Hip updrawing. (*See Fig.* 121, p. 96, which shows exercise performed in standing.)

**Secondary Exercises**

*Trunk Exercise*

Lying; Chest raising. (*See Fig.* 80, p. 79.)

## 2. PATIENT SITTING IN CHAIR

**Primary Exercises**

*Trunk Exercises*

1. Stride sitting; Trunk turning with Arm moving loosely sideways in the direction of the hands to grasp the chair back (*Fig.* 216).
2. Stride sitting; Trunk bending sideways.

**Secondary Exercises**

*Trunk Exercise*

Stride sitting (hands on thighs); Trunk bending forwards-downwards to

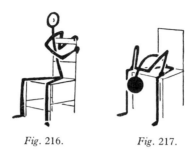

Fig. 216.          Fig. 217.

assume a modified lax stoop position (movement taken as far as possible without producing discomfort in wound area), followed by Trunk stretching. (*Fig.* 217).

## 3. PATIENT STANDING

**Primary Exercises**

*Posture and Walking*
1. General correction of posture in standing and walking.
2. Walking practice.

## 10th TO 14th POSTOPERATIVE DAY

The patient is often discharged from the ward between the 10th and 14th day.

*Remedial Aims*

PRIMARY
To redevelop the abdominal muscles, particularly the oblique and transverse groups.

SECONDARY
1. To redevelop the other trunk muscles.
2. To redevelop the muscles that support the medial longitudinal arches of the feet.
3. To re-educate neuromuscular coordination.

*Exercise Period*
30 minutes, once or twice daily.

**Primary Exercises**

*Trunk Exercises*

1. Fixed stride lying; upper Trunk bending forwards with turning and single Arm carrying across the chest. (*Fig.* 218).
2. Crook lying; Pelvis raising and turning.
3. Half lumbar rest stride standing; single Arm swinging forwards, and sideways with Trunk turning.
4. Low reach grasp standing (chair back); Hip updrawing. (*See Fig.* 121, p. 96.) which shows a different starting position.)
5. Stride standing; Trunk bending sideways.
6. Lying; high Knee raising, followed by over-pressure with the hands, and upper Trunk bending forwards. (*See Fig.* 73, p. 74.)
7. Lying; upper Trunk bending forwards with single high Knee raising. (*See Figs.* 59 and 67, pp. 70 and 73.)

**Secondary Exercises**

*Trunk Exercises*

1. Lax stoop stride sitting; Trunk stretching 'vertebra by vertebra' in different planes. (*See Fig.* 139, p. 105.)
2. Crook lying; Chest raising. (*See Fig.* 80, p. 79.)
3. Forehead rest prone lying (pillow under abdomen); single slight Leg raising backwards.
4. Neck rest stride sitting; Trunk lowering forwards.

*Leg Exercises*

5. Low reach grasp standing (chair back); inner Border raising.

*Balance Exercises*

6. Back towards standing (wall bars or wall); single Knee raising.
7. Half yard finger support side toward standing (wall bars or wall); balance walking forwards with Knee raising.

**FROM 14th POSTOPERATIVE DAY**

The exercises suggested here are of a moderately strenuous type. They are used for one to two weeks if exercise therapy is prescribed for the patient after he is discharged from the ward.

*Remedial Aims*

As for the 10th–14th postoperative day.

*Exercise Period*

30 minutes, once or twice daily.

## Primary Exercises

*Trunk Exercises*

1. Fixed stride lying; upper Trunk bending forwards with turning and single Arm carrying across the chest (*Fig.* 218).

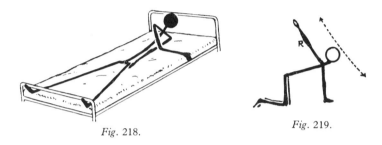

*Fig.* 218.                               *Fig.* 219.

2. Prone kneeling; slow Trunk turning with single Arm raising sideways. (*Fig.* 219.)
3. Stride standing; Trunk bending sideways.
4. Fixed crook lying; Trunk bending forwards with assistance from arms. (*See Fig.* 72, p. 74, which shows a different starting position.)
5. Fist bend fixed inclined long sitting (wall bar stool); Trunk lowering backwards through 45°. (*See Fig.* 60, p. 70.)

## Secondary Exercises

*Trunk Exercises*

1. Lax stoop back lean stride standing (heels about a footlength or more in front of wall bar upright); Trunk stretching 'vertebra by vertebra' in different planes. (*See Fig.* 139, p. 105.)
2. Neck rest crook lying; Chest raising. (*See Fig.* 80, p. 79.)
3. Forehead rest prone lying; single Leg raising backwards. The exercise may have to be modified, so that the spinal extension does not stretch the abdominal muscles unduly or cause pain.
4. Prone kneeling; Pelvis tilting forwards and backwards with Head bending backwards and forwards. (*See Fig.* 106, p. 90.)
5. Fist bend stride sitting; Trunk lowering forwards.

*Foot Exercise*

6. Standing; inner Border raising.

*Balance Exercises*
7. Balance walking forwards with opposite Knee and Arm raising.
8. Balance half standing (balance bench rib); balance walking fowards and backwards.

## 2. CHOLECYSTECTOMY

The gallbladder is removed in cases of chronic cholecystitis, with or without the presence of gallstones. Disease of the gallbladder is more common in women than in men.

### TYPES OF INCISION

The most common incision used today is the right upper paramedian incision (*Fig.* 215, p. 189). In certain cases (obese subjects, for example, where good exposure is required), Kocher's subcostal incision is used (*Fig.* 215, p. 189). This incision was employed more often in the past, before the introduction of muscle relaxing drugs in anaesthesia.

### Right Upper Paramedian Incision. (*See* p. 188.)

### Kocher's Subcostal Incision (*Fig.* 215, p. 189)

The incision begins just below the xiphoid process and extends downwards and outwards to the tip of the 9th costal cartilage, 2·5 cm below and parallel with the costal margin. All the abdominal muscles, including the lateral half of the rectus and its sheath, are divided in the same line. The 9th intercostal nerve is severed. Thus this incision produces a flaccid paralysis of certain of the fibres of the abdominal muscles, which predisposes to herniae.

### Drainage

In a straightforward cholecystectomy some form of drainage is employed for 48–72 hours. Bile secretions are drained into a Redivac vacuum bottle or a Porto-vac suction unit.

When the common bile-duct is incised and explored (for the presence of an obstructing stone), a T-tube is used to drain the common bile-duct. The tube drains into a bag attached to the patient's thigh and is usually retained for about 10 days.

## EXERCISE THERAPY

As suggested for gastrectomy (pp. 190–196). Certain modifications must be noted, as indicated here:

1. Usually intravenous therapy is not given.

2. 'Getting Up.' After cholecystectomy, when a drain is used for 48–72 hours, sitting in a chair for 10–20 minutes is usually allowed on the 1st postoperative day. Walking is encouraged when the drainage is discontinued. After cholecystectomy, with exploration of the common bile-duct (T-tube drainage into bag), the 'getting up' régime is much the same but may be a little slower.

3. Discharge from ward. After straightforward cholecystectomy the patient is usually allowed to return home between the 7th and 10th postoperative day. When the common bile-duct is explored the patient is generally discharged from the ward between the 10th and 12th postoperative day.

---

### 3. APPENDICECTOMY

Appendicectomy is performed in the treatment of acute, subacute, and chronic inflammation of the vermiform appendix. During an acute attack of appendicitis the operation may be carried out before perforation of the appendix occurs, or after perforation has occurred (when a general peritonitis will complicate the original condition). In chronic appendicitis the appendix is removed between attacks—'interval appendicectomy'.

## TYPES OF INCISION

The most common incision used in this country is the gridiron (McBurney) or muscle-splitting incision. Other incisions are Battle's pararectal incision and the right lower paramedian incision. (*See* p. 189.)

### Gridiron Incision (*Fig.* 215, p. 189)

The incision is an oblique one and runs in a downward and inward direction in the line of the fibres of the external oblique muscle. It is about 5 cm in length, with its centre at the junction of the middle and lateral thirds of a line drawn from the umbilicus to the right anterior superior iliac spine.

*Stages of Incision*

1. Incision of skin and subcutaneous tissues, down to the external oblique muscle.

2. Incision of the external oblique in the line of its fibres. Retraction of the external oblique to expose the internal oblique muscle.
3. Separation of the internal oblique and transversalis muscles in the line of their fibres.
4. Incision of the peritᵣneum.

The abdomen is closed in five stages.

**Battle's Pararectal Incision** (*Fig.* 215, p. 189)
This incision is considered to give better views, but is said to be somewhat more liable to hernia. The incision is a vertical one, sub-umbilical in position and about 5 cm in length.

**Right Lower Paramedian Incision** (*Fig.* 215, p. 189)
The incision is used when the diagnosis is uncertain, or when exploration of the lower abdomen (usually in the case of a female) is desired. *See* p. 188 for details of right upper paramedian incision.

## EXERCISE AND THE SUTURE LINE
### Gridiron Incision
Because the muscles have been split in the direction of their fibres abdominal exercises will not tend to separate the sutured muscle edges. Nevertheless, reasonable care should be shown in the choice and performance of trunk exercises throughout the postoperative phase of treatment.

### Battle's Incision and Right Lower Paramedian Incision
Both types of incision entail cutting of the anterior and posterior sheaths of the rectus muscle, which are formed by the aponeuroses of the oblique and transverse abdominal muscles. Active trunk rotation movements will therefore tend to pull more strongly on the suture line than any other form of trunk exercise. The suggestions made on p. 189 regarding choice and performance of trunk exercises in the after-treatment of gastrectomy should be followed.

## EXERCISE THERAPY
The lists of progressive exercises given here are intended to be a guide to the after-treatment of (1) Interval Appendicectomy, and (2) Appendicectomy performed for acute appendicitis before perforation has occurred. It is assumed that a gridiron incision is used.

When the pararectal or the paramedian incision is used exercise therapy is based on that suggested for gastrectomy (pp. 190–196). Progress, however, should be more rapid.

## 1st POSTOPERATIVE DAY

The patient is usually allowed to sit out in a chair for 30–45 minutes during the morning or afternoon and to walk in the ward for a short distance. While in bed he is encouraged to spend much of his time lying on his back and on the left and right sides. (*Fig.* 214, p. 186); he remains in each position for about an hour at a time. This alteration of posture assists in the ventilation of the lungs and helps to 'break' any flatulence which may be present.

*Remedial Aims*

PRIMARY
1. To prevent postoperative respiratory complications.*
2. To prevent postoperative circulatory complications.
3. To maintain the abdominal muscles, particularly the oblique and transverse groups.

SECONDARY
To maintain the other trunk muscles.

*Exercise Period*

20 minutes. In addition to this treatment session the patient will practise some of the exercises on 'little and often' lines during the day.

## Primary Exercises

*Breathing, Ankle/Foot and Leg Exercises (See* previous section, pp. 186–188.)
*Trunk Exercises*

1. Stride lying; Trunk turning with single Arm carrying across the chest (*See Fig.* 129, p. 101.)
2. Heave grasp lying (head posts of bed); Hip updrawing. (*See Fig.* 121, p. 96, which shows a different starting position.)

---

* This aim is not so important as in the treatment of conditions where the incision involves the upper abdomen (e.g. gastrectomy), because the respiratory excursion of the diaphragm is far less limited.

**Secondary Exercises**

*Trunk Exercises*

1. Lying: slight Chest raising. (*See Fig.* 80, p. 79, which shows full-range Chest raising.)
2. Crook lying; Pelvis raising. (*See Fig.* 150, p. 116.)

## 2nd–5th POSTOPERATIVE DAY

The patient spends an increasing amount of time sitting out in a chair and in walking in the ward.

*Remedial Aims*

PRIMARY

1. To prevent postoperative respiratory and circulatory complications.*
2. To maintain the abdominal muscles, particularly the oblique and transverse groups.
3. To maintain normal posture and reinstitute walking.

SECONDARY

To maintain the other trunk muscles.

*Exercise Period*

20–30 minutes daily.

**Exercises**

As after operations for inguinal hernia. (*See* pp. 205–206.)

## 6th–7th POSTOPERATIVE DAY

The stitches are removed on the 7th day. Provided that the patient's condition is satisfactory he is discharged home on the same day.

---

* These aims are achieved by the patient sitting out of bed and walking about in the ward. Breathing exercises and movements to accelerate the venous circulation through the lower limbs are therefore not necessary in the average case after the first postoperative day. In this connection it must be borne in min.d that the bulk of the appendicectomy cases fall into the younger age group, in which postoperative pulmonary and circulatory complications are less to be feared.

*Remedial Aims*

PRIMARY
To redevelop the abdominal muscles, particularly the oblique and transverse groups.

SECONDARY
1. To redevelop the other trunk muscles.
2. To re-educate neuromuscular coordination.

*Exercise Period*
30 minutes daily.

**Exercises**
As after operations for inguinal hernia. (*See* pp. 206–207.)

## FROM 7th POSTOPERATIVE DAY

The exercises suggested here are of a moderately strenuous nature. They may be used for 1–2 weeks if exercise therapy is prescribed for the patient after he has been discharged from the ward.

*Remedial Aims*
As previous section. In addition (Secondary): To promote generalized activity.

*Exercise Period*
30 minutes daily.

**Exercises**
As after operations for inguinal hernia. (*See* pp. 208–209.)

## 4. OPERATIONS FOR INGUINAL HERNIA

### DEFENCE MECHANISM OF INGUINAL CANAL
The inguinal canal constitutes a weak area in the abdominal wall. During a temporary increase in intra-abdominal pressure, such as occurs, for example, in coughing and defaecation, there is a tendency for the abdominal viscera to

be forced into the canal. The canal possesses an efficient defence mechanism against this occurrence:

## Shutter Action

The muscles of the inguinal region 'react to strain in the following manner: (1) Contraction of the external oblique narrows the gap in the external ring. (2) Associated tightening of the rectus sheath and the underlying muscle forms a firm foundation for the remaining actions. (3) Straightening of the arched conjoint tendon diminishes the interval between it and the inguinal ligament, but a weakened triangular area persists with its base in the region of the emerging cord at the external ring, due to the tendinous segment of conjoint tendon. Recurrent herniae are common at this site and care should be taken at operation to repair this portion adequately. (4) Lateral and upward movement of the U-shaped internal ring tightens the fascia transversalis. (5) Finally, there is blockage of the inguinal canal by the bulk of the cremaster muscle which is pulled upwards on contraction' (Macfarlane and Thomas, 1977).

## Valvular Mechanism

The obliquity of the canal (which to some extent constitutes a valvular mechanism) is an additional safeguard. Increased intra-abdominal pressure apposes firmly the posterior and anterior walls of the canal. Opposite the area of greatest weakness in the posterior wall (the deep inguinal ring) is placed the strongest part of the abdominal wall: the internal oblique fibres and the aponeurosis of the external oblique.

## INGUINAL HERNIA

An inguinal hernia results when the mechanism of the inguinal canal fails and the abdominal viscera escape through the deep inguinal ring, the inguinal canal, and the superficial inguinal ring, to reach sometimes the scrotum or labium majus. The escaped viscera are contained in a sac which is composed of peritoneum and extraperitoneal tissue.

The hernial sac descends within the coverings of the spermatic cord in the male; its contents may include omentum, bowel, fluid, or loose bodies (from omentum). The most common contents are omentum and small intestine.

Failure of the inguinal mechanism may be the result of irregularities in the development of the contents of the canal (congenital hernia). It may also be due to loss of the shutter action from the hypotonus of age or debility (acquired hernia). 'In the most frequent type, the hernia passes down the inguinal canal. For this reason it is referred to as "oblique inguinal hernia". Weakness of the abdominal musculature may, however, allow the abdominal contents to be extruded at the other weak area of the inguinal region—opposite the subcutaneous (superficial) inguinal ring. This variety, which does not traverse the full length of the canal, is referred to as "direct inguinal hernia" ' (Beesly and Johnson, 1939).

Oblique inguinal hernia may develop at any age, but 'it most commonly appears first in infancy, youth or early adult life. It is commoner in males than in females' (Aird, 1957a).

## OBLIQUE INGUINAL HERNIA: OPERATIVE PROCEDURES

In general, two main types of operative treatment for oblique inguinal hernia may be recognized. (1) Simple herniotomy, or complete removal of the sac. This is the method of choice in infants, children and young fit adults, where the hernia is generally congenital and the secondary changes in the inguinal canal still revisable. (2) Excision of the hernial sac, followed by repair of the inguinal canal. This is usually indicated in the older age group (where the abdominal musculature is of poor quality) and in the case of recurrent hernias.

### Simple Herniotomy

An incision is made about a finger's breadth above and parallel to the medial two-thirds of the inguinal ligament, so as to expose the aponeurosis of the external oblique muscle. (*See Fig.* 215, p. 189.) The margin of the superficial inguinal ring is defined and the cord is isolated. The aponeurosis of the external oblique is divided from the subcutaneous ring along the line of the inguinal canal. The coverings of the cord are then divided and the sac identified. The sac is transfixed at its neck, ligated and removed. The wound is closed in three stages.

### Excision of Sac with Repair of Canal

After excision of the hernial sac a variety of methods may be used to repair the inguinal canal. The Bassini operation is summarized here.

*Bassini Procedure*

The operation aims at strengthening the whole of the potentially weak posterior wall of the inguinal canal by suturing the internal oblique muscle and the conjoint tendon to the inguinal ligament, behind the spermatic cord. This method has been much criticized, and Aird (1957b) states that it should be used 'only if the conjoint tendon and inguinal ligament lie close together and parallel, so that they may be apposed without tension'. If they are brought together under tension, the conjoint tendon may tear, thus losing the desired effect. A further criticism levelled at the Bassini operation is that it is said to interfere with the shutter mechanism of the canal.


## ABDOMINAL EXERCISES FOLLOWING OPERATIONS FOR INGUINAL HERNIA

The scope of abdominal exercises depends on the type of operative procedure which has been performed.


### After Simple Herniotomy

Abdominal exercises assist in the functional recovery of the inguinal mechanism (p. 202), and so help to prevent a recurrence of the hernia.


*Exercise and the Suture Line*

Because the aponeurosis of the external oblique muscle is divided in the line of its fibres, abdominal exercises will not tend to separate the sutured edges. Reasonable care should be taken, however, in the choice and performance of trunk exercises throughout the postoperative phase of treatment.


### After Excision of Hernial Sac, with Repair by Bassini Operation

Abdominal exercises help to restore the strength of the abdominal muscles, and so assist in the recovery of the valvular aspect of the inguinal mechanism (p. 202). It is debatable if the exercises can assist in the functional recovery of the shutter mechanism of the canal; theoretically, this has been obliterated by the repair process. In practice, however, it may be doubted if such function has been completely replaced.


*Exercise and the Suture Line*

Much the same attitude towards trunk exercises may be taken as previously suggested. From experience it would appear that the repair procedures do not necessitate a more conservative approach to exercise therapy.


## EXERCISE THERAPY

The lists of progressive exercises given here are intended to be a guide to the after treatment of (*a*) Simple herniotomy, and (*b*) Excision of hernial sac, with repair of inguinal canal by Bassini operation.

## FIRST 3 POSTOPERATIVE DAYS

On the 1st postoperative day the patient is generally allowed to sit in a chair for about 30–45 minutes and to walk a little in the ward. The amount of sitting and walking is gradually increased over the 3 days.

When resting in bed the patient should spend some of his time lying flat on his back and on the left and right sides (*Fig.* 214, p. 186); he should remain in each position for about an hour at a time. This alteration of posture assists in the ventilation of the lungs and helps to 'break' any flatulence which may be present.

### *Remedial Aims*

PRIMARY
1. To prevent postoperative respiratory and circulatory complications.
2. To maintain the abdominal muscles, particularly the oblique and transverse groups.
3. To maintain the mobility of the hip joint of the affected side.

SECONDARY
To maintain the other trunk muscles.

### *Exercise Period*

20–30 minutes daily. In addition to this treatment session the patient will practise some of the exercises on 'little and often' lines throughout the day.

### Primary Exercises

*Breathing, Ankle/Foot and Leg Exercises* (*see* previous section, pp. 186–188)

TRUNK EXERCISES
1. Stride lying; Trunk turning with single Arm carrying across the chest. (*See Fig.* 129, p. 101.)
2. Crook lying (hand on abdomen); Abdominal contractions.
3. Lying; Head bending forwards with single slight Knee raising.
4. Lying (hands grasping sides of mattress); Hip updrawing. (*See Fig.* 121, p. 96, which shows a different starting position.)

HIP EXERCISES
5. Lying; single Knee raising (of affected side), gradually increasing range of movement.
6. Lying; single Leg carrying sideways.

**Secondary Exercises**

TRUNK EXERCISES

7. Lying; slight Chest raising.(*See Fig.* 80, p. 79, which shows full-range Chest raising.)
8. Crook lying; Pelvis raising. (*See Fig.* 150, p. 116.)

## 4th–7th POSTOPERATIVE DAY

The patient spends an increasing amount of time sitting in a chair and walking about in the ward. The stitches are removed on the 7th postoperative day. (Absorbable cutaneous sutures are sometimes used.) The patient is warned not to attempt to lift any heavy object. Before being discharged home he should be given some elementary instruction in the correct techniques of lifting and carrying.

*Remedial Aims*

PRIMARY

1. To prevent postoperative respiratory and circulatory complications.*
2. To maintain the abdominal muscles, particularly the oblique and transverse groups.
3. To maintain normal posture and reinstate good walking habits.

SECONDARY

To maintain the other trunk muscles.

*Exercise Period*

30 minutes daily.

## 1. PATIENT LYING ON BED

**Primary Exercises**

*Trunk Exercises*

1. Stride lying; Trunk turning with Head bending forwards and single Arm carrying across the chest. (*See Fig.* 129, p. 101.)
1. Crook lying (hands grasping sides of mattress); slow Knee swinging from side to side. (*See Fig.* 128, p. 100.)
3. Lying (hands grasping sides of mattress); Hip updrawing. (*See Fig.* 121, p. 96, which shows the exercise in standing.)

---

* These aims are achieved by the patient sitting out of bed and walking about in the ward. Breathing exercises and movements to accelerate the venous circulation through the lower limbs are therefore not necessary in the average case after the 3rd postoperative day.

4. Lying; Head bending forwards with single Knee raising.
5. Lying (hands grasping sides of mattress); upper Trunk bending forwards with assistance from arms.
6. Crook lying; Pelvis tilting forwards and backwards (range of forward tilt being restricted). (*See Figs.* 68 and 79, pp. 73 and 79.)

## Secondary Exercises
*Trunk Exercises*
1. Crook lying; slight Chest raising. (*See Fig.* 80, p. 79, which shows full-range Chest raising.)

## 2. PATIENT SITTING IN CHAIR
### Primary Exercises
*Trunk Exercises*
1. Stride sitting; Trunk turning with Arm moving loosely sideways in the direction of the turning to grasp the chair back. (*See Fig.* 216, p. 193.)
2. Stride sitting; Trunk bending sideways.

## Secondary Exercises
1. Stride sitting (hands on thighs); Trunk bending forwards-downwards to assume a modified lax stoop position (movement taken as far as possible without producing discomfort in wound area), followed by Trunk stretching 'vertebra by vertebra'. (*See Fig.* 217, p. 193.)

## 3. PATIENT STANDING
### Primary Exercises
*Check on Posture and Walking*
1. General correction of posture in standing and walking.
2. Walking practice.

## FROM 7th POSTOPERATIVE DAY

The exercises suggested here are of a moderately strenuous type. They may be used for 1–2 weeks if exercise therapy is prescribed for the patient after he has been discharged from the ward.

*Remedial Aims*

PRIMARY
1. To redevelop the abdominal muscles, particularly the oblique and transverse groups.
2. To educate the patient in the correct technique of lifting and carrying heavy objects.

SECONDARY
1. To redevelop the other trunk muscles.
2. To re-educate neuromuscular coordination.

*Exercise Period*
30 minutes daily.

## Primary Exercises

*Trunk Exercises*
1. Fixed stride lying; upper Trunk bending forwards with turning and single Arm carrying across the chest. (*See Fig.* 218, p. 195.)
2. Prone kneeling; slow Trunk turning with single Arm raising sideways.
3. Half lumbar rest stride standing; single Arm swinging forwards, and sideways with Trunk turning.
4. Low reach grasp standing (chair back); Hip updrawing. (*See Fig.* 121, p. 96.)
5. Lying; Trunk bending sideways with single Leg carrying sideways to the same side.
6. Stride standing; Trunk bending sideways.
7. Lying; high Knee raising, followed by over-pressure with the hands, and upper Trunk bending forwards. (*See Fig.* 73, p. 74.)
8. Lying; upper Trunk bending forwards with single high Knee raising. (*See Figs.* 59 and 67, pp. 70 and 73.)

*Education in Lifting*
9. Practice in correct technique of lifting and carrying heavy objects. (*Fig.* 220).

## Secondary Exercises

*Trunk Exercises*
1. Lax stoop back lean stride standing (heels about a foot-length in front of wall bar upright); Trunk stretching 'vertebra by vertebra' in different planes. (*See Fig.* 139, p. 105.)
2. Crook lying; Chest raising. (*See Fig.* 80, p. 79.)

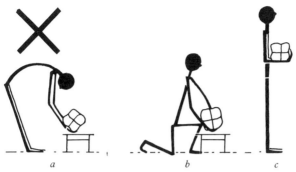

*Fig.* 220. *a,* Incorrect lifting technique. *b,* Correct lifting technique. Note straight back, position of legs and feet (giving stable base), and firm hold on object lifted. *c,* Correct carrying posture: object held securely and close to body, vision unobstructed.

### Balance Exercises

3. Balance walking forwards and backwards with Knee raising.
4. Balance walking fowards with opposite Knee and Arm raising.

## 5. FEMORAL AND UMBILICAL HERNIAE

### FEMORAL HERNIA

A femoral hernia consists of a downward extension of peritoneum through the femoral canal. Usually the hernia is not very large; as a rule the sac contains omentum.

Femoral hernia is commoner in women than in men. This is said to be because the inguinal ligament makes a wider angle with the pubis in the female, and pregnancies increase intra-abdominal pressure.

Men who suffer from this condition usually follow 'stooping' occupations: bakers, stokers and gardeners.

### Surgical Treatment

An operation is performed unless there is some definite contra-indication. The sac is ligated and the femoral canal closed. Two main types of procedure are employed, the high operation and the low operation.

#### High Operation

An incision is made, similar to that described for simple inguinal herniotomy (p. 203), above and parallel to the medial two-thirds of the inguinal ligament. The external oblique aponeurosis is divided and the posterior wall of the inguinal canal exposed; the protuberance of peritoneum which forms the hernia can then be drawn out of the femoral canal from above.

*Low Operation*

A vertical incision, 5–7·5 cm in length, is made over the hernial protuberance. The sac is exposed and dealt with from below.

In both operations the hernial sac is cleared of its coverings, opened, explored, and the contents (if any) returned to the general peritoneal cavity. The pectineal fascia is sutured to the under-surface of the inguinal ligament. This closes the femoral canal.

**Postoperative Exercise Therapy**

As for operations for inguinal hernia (pp. 205–209). Exercises for the hip of the affected side are important during the first few postoperative days.

## UMBILICAL HERNIA

An umbilical hernia consists of a protrusion of the abdominal contents through the umbilicus. If the protrusion occurs close to the umbilicus the condition is known as a 'para-umbilical hernia'.

Adult umbilical hernia occurs almost exclusively in obese women at the end of the child-bearing period. The hernia is probably the effect of increased intra-abdominal pressure (pregnancies, omental adiposity, bronchitis) on the umbilical cicatrix or the linea alba. The hernia sometimes reaches a huge size. It contains usually omentum and sometimes transverse colon and small intestine as well.

**Surgical Treatment**

The hernia is treated by operation. Before operation an attempt is often made to reduce the patient's weight by dietetic means.

A transverse elliptical incision is made which outlines the hernial protrusion; it is deepened through the fat until the stretched linea alba is exposed. The sac is defined and opened. Protruding bowel is returned to the general peritoneal cavity; omentum may be widely excised to reduce the volume of the abdominal contents; the sac is then ligated at the neck and excised.

The stretched linea alba is sutured transversely with two rows of stitches, so that the flaps overlap; the subcutaneous tissues and the skin are then sutured.

**Exercise Therapy**

*After Repair of a Small Umbilical Hernia*

As after operations for inguinal hernia (pp. 205–209.)

*After Repair of a Large Umbilical Hernia*

The patient remains in the ward for about 10 days. Usually she is allowed to sit in a chair on the 1st or 2nd postoperative day for 15–20 minutes. The time of sitting out and walking is gradually increased. The stitches are generally removed on the 10th day.

Great care must be taken in exercising the abdominal muscles, because the tissues are of poor quality and any excessive strain may break down the repair and cause reherniation. The same types of abdominal exercises are used as described for simple inguinal herniotomy (pp. 205–209), but the time suggested for starting the exercises in sitting and standing must be delayed. In addition, some of the stronger abdominal exercises must be omitted in the early stages of treatment.

An abdominal belt or corset is worn when the patient is allowed out of bed. She must wear it when she first sits out, as well as when standing and walking.

## REFERENCES

Aird I. (1957a) *A Companion in Surgical Studies*, 2nd ed. Edinburgh, Livingstone, p. 527.
Aird I. (1957b) *Ibid.* p. 646.
Ballinger W. F. and Drapanas T. (1972) *Practice of Surgery*. St Louis, Mosby, pp. 166–7.
Beesly L. and Johnson T. B. (1939) *Manual of Surgical Anatomy*, 5th ed. London, Oxford University Press, p. 340.
Bendixen H. H. (1965) *Respiratory Care*. St Louis, Mosby.
Macfarlane D. A. and Thomas L. P. (1977) *Textbook of Surgery*, 4th ed. Edinburgh, Churchill Livingstone, pp. 240–1.

# 20. Intervertebral disc lesions of the lumbar spine

When the annulus fibrosus of the intervertebral disc remains intact, but bulges posteriorly, the patient may complain of low back pain. When, however, the annulus ruptures and a prolapse of the nucleus pulposus occurs, the prolapse may impinge on a lumbar nerve root and cause sciatica.

Conservative treatment will be sufficient for most disc lesions. Surgical treatment will be required for a small percentage of patients in whom the prolapse cannot be warded off the nerve root.

## CONSERVATIVE TREATMENT

Conservative treatment consists of:

1. *Bed rest* in the supine position on a rigid mattress for one to three weeks. Traction may be applied to the lower limbs (skin extension) or to the pelvis by means of a well-padded pelvic band. If traction is used the foot end of the bed is elevated.

2. *Intermittent spinal traction.* This is generally carried out in the physiotherapy department. The method of application will depend on the patient's condition and the clinical judgement of the therapist.

3. *Manipulation.* On some occasions this will be carried out by the orthopaedic surgeon, with or without a general anaesthetic. On other occasions manipulation will be performed by a physiotherapist skilled in passive mobilization techniques.

4. *Spinal support*: plaster-of-Paris jacket, surgical brace or belt. All these supports are individually made and fitted.

*Exercise therapy* is often used in association with these conservative measures. It should be noted that some surgeons do not allow trunk exercises when bed rest is prescribed (*see* Programme 1, p. 213).

## SURGICAL TREATMENT

Surgical treatment consists of the removal of the prolapsed portion of the intervertebral disc. Exercise therapy is used in the postoperative phase of recovery, as described on pp. 215–220.

## EXERCISE THERAPY WHEN CONSERVATIVE TREATMENT IS USED

The exercise programmes outlined in this section have been arranged for use when bed rest, with or without traction, is used. Programme 2 may be modified for use when other conservative measures are employed, e.g. spinal support by plaster-of-Paris jacket or surgical brace. The emphasis of treatment is then on strengthening the muscles of the spine, particularly the extensors.

### PROGRAMME 1: WHEN BED REST, WITH OR WITHOUT TRACTION, IS USED

*Remedial Aims*

PRIMARY

1. To maintain the strength of the muscles and the mobility of the joints of the lower limbs within the limits imposed by the patient's condition and the method of immobilization used.
2. To maintain the strength of the muscles and the mobility of the shoulder joints and joints of the shoulder girdle.
3. To prevent possible respiratory and circulatory complications during the period of immobilization.

*Exercise Period*

Initially, 10–15 minutes, twice daily. Supervised exercise periods are replaced as soon as possible by self-care practice on 'little and often' lines.

### Examples of Primary Exercises

*Leg Exercises*

1. Lying; single and double Quadriceps contractions.
2. Lying; single and double Gluteal contractions.
3. Lying; single and double Ankle bending.
4. Lying; (*a*) single and double Foot turning inwards, (*b*) single and double Foot turning outwards.
5. Lying; single Foot circling.
6. Lying; single small range Knee raising with heel in contact with supporting surface (i.e. flexion of each hip and knee through a 'comfortable' range, not exceeding 15° of hip flexion).

*Shoulder and Shoulder girdle Exercises*

7. Heave lying; inward and outward rotation of shoulder joints.

8. Lying; Shoulder rounding and bracing.
9. Lying; Shoulder shrugging.

*Breathing Exercises*

10. Lying (hands on sides of lower chest); lower lateral Costal breathing.
11. Lying (hand on upper abdomen); Diaphragmatic breathing.

## PROGRAMME 2: WHEN SYMPTOMS HAVE SUBSIDED AND TRACTION, IF USED, IS DISCONTINUED

The patient rests in bed for a day or so and then progresses to short periods of sitting, standing and walking; it is important that a chair of suitable height and design is used. The emphasis of exercise treatment is on (*a*) strengthening the main trunk muscles, particularly the extensors; and (*b*) promoting the mobility of the thoracolumbar spine and knee joints. If spinal flexion is allowed by the surgeon it is best carried out in side-lying.

### Examples of Primary Exercises

*Back Exercises*

1. Lying; Chest raising. (*See Fig.* 80, p. 79.)
2. Prone lying; Shoulder bracing.
3. Forearm support prone lying; Trunk bending backwards with assistance from arms. (*See Fig.* 37*a*, p. 51.)
4. Prone lying (arms behind back, fingers clasped); Trunk bending backwards with Arm raising backwards.
5. Lying; opposite Arm and Leg downpressing.

*Abdominal Exercise*

6. Lying; Head bending forwards.

*Rotation Exercises*

7. Stride lying; small range Trunk turning (i.e. raising one shoulder well off the bed).
8. Lying (hands grasping sides of bed); Pelvis turning from side to side.

*Lateral Flexion Exercise*

9. Stride lying; Trunk bending sideways.

*Knee Exercise*

10. Prone lying; alternate Knee bending.

## Postural Training

The patient must be made aware of the importance of maintaining a sound posture, especially when standing and sitting. A full-length mirror is of great value in this respect. The need to guard against flexion stresses of the spine (and in some instances to prevent flexion taking place) must also be emphasized.

## Technique of Lifting and Back Care

It is essential to give instruction in correct lifting and carrying techniques, with particular reference to the patient's occupation. (*See Fig.* 220, p. 209.)

---

## EXERCISE THERAPY WHEN SURGICAL TREATMENT IS USED

---

The patient is returned from the operating theatre in a side-lying position. Side-lying is maintained for at least 24 hours, the position being changed from right to left, and vice versa, at regular 2-hour intervals. A firm pillow is positioned between the knees.

A well-padded adhesive dressing is used over the incision area. Intravenous therapy is sometimes used for a day or so. In certain instances a Redivac wound drain is employed for up to 48 hours.

About the 2nd postoperative day the patient is encouraged to take up a back-lying position, provided that it does not give rise to pain and discomfort. From then on the patient's resting posture varies between back-lying and side-lying.

During this initial postoperative period the patient is encouraged to move freely in bed and to carry out simple exercises to prevent postoperative respiratory and circulatory complications.

*Sitting out of Bed*

The patient is allowed to sit out in a suitable chair (at the bedside) for short periods between the 2nd and 5th postoperative day. It is important that a chair of correct height and design is used.

*Spinal Flexion*

Opinion varies among orthopaedic surgeons as to when simple flexion movements of the thoracolumbar spine should be started. Some allow flexion in side-lying about the 6th postoperative day, while others delay this until the sutures have been removed (10th or 12th postoperative day). Others prohibit specific flexion movements.

*After Sutures have been Removed*

The patient is discharged home when the sutures have been removed; he attends the hospital for exercise therapy for 4–6 weeks, depending on his occupation.

## PROGRAMME 1: FIRST 2 POSTOPERATIVE DAYS

*Remedial Aims*

PRIMARY

1. To prevent postoperative respiratory complications. (*See* pp. 184–185.)
2. To accelerate the circulation through the veins of the lower limbs and pelvis. (*See* p. 187.)

*Exercise Period*

10 minutes, two or three times daily.

### Primary Exercises

Breathing exercises, particularly unilateral Apical and lower lateral Costal breathing; foot and ankle exercises, with emphasis on dorsiflexion movements; and small range flexion and extension of hip and knee (in side-lying this is confined to the uppermost limb).

## PROGRAMME 2: 3rd TO 10th OR 12th POSTOPERATIVE DAY WHEN SUTURES ARE REMOVED

*Remedial Aims*

PRIMARY

As in previous section. In addition: To strengthen the muscles of the thoracolumbar spine, particularly the extensors.

*Exercise Period*

15–20 minutes, twice daily.

### Primary Exercises

*Back Exercises*

1. Lying; slight Chest raising. (*See Fig.* 80, p. 79, which shows a full range movement.)
2. Lying; opposite Arm and Leg downpressing.
3. Prone lying; Shoulder bracing with Arm raising backwards.

4. Forearm support prone lying; small range Trunk bending backwards with assistance from arms. (*See Fig.* 37a, p. 51.)
5. Prone lying; small range single Leg raising backwards.
6. Prone lying (arms behind back, fingers clasped); Trunk bending backwards with Arm raising backwards.

*Abdominal (Static) Exercise*

7. Lying; Head bending forwards.

*Breathing and Leg Exercises*

8. Breathing, foot, ankle, and static Quadriceps exercises.
9. Lying; single Hip and Knee flexion.
10. Lying; single and double Gluteal contractions.
11. Prone lying; alternate Knee bending.

*N.B.* (1) From about the 5th postoperative day the patient will be encouraged to carry out some simple trunk movements in the erect position. For example: (*a*) lateral flexion movements of the thoracolumbar spine in stride standing, (*b*) gentle small range trunk rotation in the same starting position. In addition, in standing, the patient will be encouraged to exercise the quadriceps and gluteal muscle groups by small range flexion and extension movements of hips and knees.

(2) In the early stages of standing and walking a Rollator (adjusted to the patient's height) can be used effectively to provide both stability and confidence.

## PROGRAMME 3: FROM 10th OR 12th POSTOPERATIVE DAY FOR A PERIOD OF 2 WEEKS

*Remedial Aims*

PRIMARY

1. To strengthen the muscles of the thoracolumbar spine, particularly the extensors.
2. To increase the mobility of the joints of the thoracolumbar spine.
3. To teach sound postural habits and provide instruction in back care.

*Exercise Period*

30 minutes, once daily. Extra time should be allowed if pool therapy is used.

**Primary Exercises**

*Back Exercises*

1. Lying; Chest raising. (*See Fig.* 80, p. 79.)
2. Stride lying or lying; Pelvis raising (bridging). (*See Fig.* 31*b*, p. 47.)
3. Prone lying; Trunk bending backwards with Arm turning outwards. (*See Fig.* 85, p. 81.)
4. Prone lying; single Leg raising backwards.

*Abdominal Exercise*

*5. Lying; upper Trunk bending forwards with assistance from arms.

*Combined Flexion and Extension Exercises*

*6. Side lying; slow high Knee raising with or without Trunk bending forwards, followed by Trunk bending backwards with Leg stretching and carrying backwards. (*See Fig.* 99, p. 86.)
*7. Prone kneeling; Pelvis tilting forwards and backwards with Head bending backwards and forwards. (*See Fig.* 106, p. 90.)

*Rotation Exercises*

8. Stride lying; Trunk turning with single Arm carrying across the chest. (*See Fig.* 129, p. 101.)
9. Yard (palms on floor) crook lying; Knee lowering from side to side. (*See Fig.* 128, p. 100, which shows the movement performed as a swinging action.)

*Lateral Flexion Exercises*

10. Stride lying; Trunk bending from side to side.
11. Lying (hands grasping sides of mat); Hip updrawing. (*See Fig.* 121, p. 96, which shows the exercise performed in standing.)

**Postural Training**

The patient should be made aware of the importance of maintaining a sound posture at all times, particularly when at work. The need to guard against flexion stresses of the spine must be emphasized.

**Back Care**

It is important to give adequate instruction in correct lifting and carrying techniques, with particular reference to the patient's occupation.

---

* Used if spinal flexion is allowed.

## PROGRAMME 4: FROM 4th TO 6th WEEK OF RECOVERY

*Remedial Aims*

As in previous section.


*Exercise Period*

30 minutes, once daily. Extra time should be allowed if pool therapy is used.

*N.B.* Progressive circuit training forms a useful alternative to the exercises suggested here. In addition, in the later stages of recovery, a pre-work circuit designed to simulate normal working stresses (p. 251) can be used. Recreational therapy, in the form of modified volley ball and basket ball, can also be used.


### Primary Exercises

*Back Exercises*

1. High reach grasp lying (wall bars: hands grasping 5th or 6th bar from floor); spanning. (*See Fig.* 81, p. 80.)
2. Prone lying; Trunk bending backwards with Arm turning outwards and single Leg raising backwards. (*See Fig.* 5, p. 10.)
3. Fist bend fixed prone lying; Trunk bending backwards.
4. Fist bend fixed prone lying; Trunk bending backwards with turning. (*See Fig.* 138, p. 105, which shows a stronger version of the exercise.)


*Abdominal Exercises*

*5. Fixed crook lying; upper Trunk bending forwards with palms of hands resting on mat.
*6. Crook lying; small range Knee raising.


*Combined Flexion and Extension Exercise*

*7. Prone kneeling; single high Knee raising with Head bending forwards, followed by Leg stretching and raising backwards with Head bending backwards, and return to starting position. (*See Fig.* 98, p. 86.)


*Rotation Exercises*

8. Turn prone kneeling (one arm bent across chest); Trunk turning with single Arm raising sideways. (*See Fig.* 132, p. 102, which shows the exercise performed as a mobility exercise.)

---

* Used if spinal flexion is allowed.

9. Yard (palms on floor) half crook half vertical leg lift lying; Leg lowering sideways. (*See Fig.* 130, p. 101.)

*Lateral Flexion Exercise*

10. Wing fixed side towards standing (wall bars); Trunk bending sideways towards the bars, and bending away from the bars. (*See Fig.* 125, p. 99, which shows an advanced mobilizing form of the exercise.)

## REFERENCES

Adams J. C. (1980) *Standard Orthopaedic Operations*, 2nd ed. Edinburgh, Churchill Livingstone, pp. 108–114.
Edmonson A. S. and Crenshaw A. H. (ed.) (1980) *Campbell's Operative Orthopaedics*, Vol. 2, 6th ed. St Louis, Mosby, pp. 2107–2114.

# 21. Total hip replacement

Total hip replacement is widely used today in the surgical treatment of such conditions as osteo- and rheumatoid arthritis, associated not only with pain and discomfort but with severe restriction of joint movement and loss of function. The procedure is also used following severe trauma of the hip joint associated with specific damage to the acetabulum.

In recent years some orthopaedic surgeons have used total hip replacement successfully to restore movement in old joint conditions which have resulted in obliteration of the joint surfaces, e.g. bony ankylosis of the joint following acute suppurative arthritis or tuberculosis in childhood. Total hip replacement is often employed when previous hip surgery has proved unsuccessful. For example, after partial or hemi-arthroplasty.

In general, total hip replacement is confined to patients in the older age group. When used for younger patients it is usually because of severe trauma to the hip or a crippling rheumatoid condition. Commenting on this, Longton (1982) states: 'The strength of a man-made prosthesis necessarily fails with stress and use. Prostheses of at least reasonable durability are feasible, and hip prostheses have given service for 20 years or so—usually in the elderly, frail, or crippled. The story may prove different if the appliances are used in young, heavy, active individuals.'

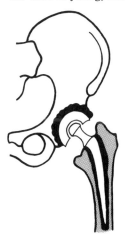

*Fig.* 221. Total replacement of the hip joint with a low friction type of prosthesis: high density polyethylene cup and stainless steel femoral component. Fixation is by methacrylate cement. (Illustration reproduced from *Textbook of Surgery*, 4th ed., by kind permission of the editors, David A. Macfarlane FRCS and Lewis P. Thomas FRCS, and the publishers, Churchill Livingstone.)

221

The low friction Charnley hip prosthesis (*Fig.* 221) is the most widely used of the many different types of prostheses designed for total hip replacement. It employs a femoral component of either stainless steel or cobalt–chrome alloy and a high-density polyethylene acetabulum. The femoral head is small, 22·25 mm in diameter. Both the femoral stem and acetabular component are cemented in position by a polymerizing plastic cement, such as methyl methacrylate.

The artificial weight-bearing surfaces between metal and polyethylene provide low friction areas capable of withstanding immense forces of many times the body-weight. A strain gauge inserted in a hip prosthesis has revealed that 'forces of at least four times the total body-weight may pass through such a joint in taking a single walking step' (Longton, 1973).

For patients who are heavier than normal (over 80 kg in weight) a heavy duty prosthesis, with a thicker stem, is employed.

## PREOPERATIVE ASSESSMENT

Normally the patient is admitted to hospital a few days before the operation is to be performed. This ensures that there is adequate time for the various preoperative tests and procedures to be carried out, e.g. cross-matching of blood and X-ray examination. The period also gives the therapist an opportunity of making a careful assessment of the patient's function, establishing a good rapport, and gauging his future physical potential with regard to age and general condition. In this respect an understanding of the patient's past medical history is essential.

In making an assessment the therapist will concentrate on: (*a*) range of movement of the joints of the lower limbs of both the affected and sound sides with particular reference to possible joint deformities and inequality between the lengths of the limbs; (*b*) effectiveness of the muscles controlling these joints; (*c*) range of movement of the lumbar spine; and (*d*) ability of the upper limbs to handle and control walking aids. The special problems of the elderly with regard to impairment of sight, hearing and general co-ordination must also be borne in mind.

## PREOPERATIVE EXERCISE THERAPY

*Respiratory Function*

As most patients for hip arthroplasty are in the older age group, and the operation itself is a major and lengthy procedure, it is vital that every effort is made to improve respiratory function. Many patients are totally unaware of their poor respiratory levels, particularly those who have been habitual smokers.

Correct breathing techniques are taught as soon as possible after the patient is admitted to the ward and continued on a regular basis until he is discharged home. Smoking is not allowed for 48 hours before the operation; many patients resent this bitterly, and have to be handled with considerable firmness by both nursing and therapy staff. After the operation smoking is discouraged; often this presents fewer difficulties than would have been expected; patients come to realize the value of their improved respiratory function.

The breathing exercises used are those recommended in the section dealing with postoperative respiratory exercises, pp. 186–187. Because of the lack of hip mobility the half lying position is used in place of crook lying.

Although the bilateral approach to costal breathing is employed the patient must also be taught unilateral breathing techniques. Unilateral exercises are important in the early postoperative phase of treatment when one of the patient's arms will be used for intravenous therapy.

*Rehearsing Position of Immobilization*

It is necessary to explain and demonstrate the position of immobilization which the patient will be required to maintain immediately after surgery. Salient points include: (*a*) Abduction of the affected hip joint to 20° (some surgeons prefer bilateral hip abduction); and (*b*) Avoidance of lateral rotation of the affected hip. 'Big toe pointing towards the ceiling . . . ' is a useful hint in this connection.

*Bridging*

A modified bridging manœuvre (used for toilet purposes and other nursing procedures) is taught with the sound leg flexed at hip and knee and the affected limb well supported by the therapist or nurse (*see* p. 47). The use of a correctly adjusted 'monkey' chain or strap can be of considerable assistance in stabilizing the body during the bridging movement.

Bridging, as described here, needs to be practised carefully by the patient. This will help to minimize the risk of possible dislocation of the prosthesis when a bed-pan is used in the early phase of postoperative care.

## PREOPERATIVE EXERCISE PROGRAMME

A simple programme of exercises is started as soon as possible after admission. It aims at (*a*) improving respiratory function, (*b*) maintaining the strength of the quadriceps and gluteal muscle groups, (*c*) accelerating the venous circulation through the veins of the lower limbs and pelvis, and (*d*) improving the mobility of the joints of the lower limbs. The programme should also include suitable exercises to strengthen the muscles of the upper limbs and shoulder girdle in preparation for the use of walking aids.

When possible, it is advisable to measure the patient for the appropriate walking aid—generally elbow crutches, but sometimes a walking frame—and to give instruction in their correct use. The patient should then be encouraged to walk freely in the ward with the help of his specific aid.

## Examples of Preoperative Exercises

1. Half lying; breathing exercises (both unilateral and bilateral). (*See* pp. 109–110.)
2. Half lying; single and double Quadriceps contractions.
3. Half lying; single and double Gluteal contractions.
4. Half lying; single and double Ankle bending.
5. Half lying; alternate Ankle bending and stretching.
6. Lying; single Knee raising with heel in contact with supporting surface, followed by Leg downpressing: sound limb only.
7. Lying; same exercise as above, but confined to affected limb. Therapist encourages the widest range of movement possible. In practical terms only a few degrees of true hip flexion may be possible.
8. Lying; single and double Hip abduction. At the affected hip movement may be limited to a few degrees.
9. Bend (fists on chest) stride lying; Elbow circling backwards.
10. Stride lying; single Arm raising forwards-upwards and rhythmical pressing in final position.
11. Standing; correction of faulty posture as far as possible. The use of a posture mirror is an advantage in giving this form of instruction. It increases the patient's awareness of his faulty stance.

## POSTOPERATIVE TREATMENT

When the patient is returned to the ward from the recovery room he is placed on the bed in a modified lying position (trunk raised slightly) with either the affected leg, or both legs, abducted to 20°. The abducted position is used to ensure the stability of the prosthesis in the new acetabulum.

A variety of methods of fixation and support is used to maintain the abducted position of the hips. For example: (*a*) Triangular foam wedge with wide base positioned between ankles; (*b*) Individual foam gutter trough or troughs; (*c*) Individual thigh slings attached to the sides of the bed; (*d*) Ankle 'gaiters' attached to a horizontal strut; (*e*) Pillow 'mound' positioned between the knees; and (*f*) Hamilton–Russell traction arranged to provide positive abduction for the affected limb.

Intravenous therapy will be used for a day or so: the dorsum of one of the hands is generally used for this purpose. A vacuum drain (Porto Vac or Redivac) is used for approximately 24 hours to drain the wound area. A bed cradle is in position to protect the affected limb from the weight of the bedclothes.

## POSTOPERATIVE EXERCISE THERAPY

Individual surgeons have established their own particular régimes of rehabilitative treatment following total hip replacement. Some consider that it is only necessary to give practice in standing and walking; others stress the importance of using simple bed exercises as a preliminary to walking training.

From practical experience the authors consider that the latter régime has much to commend it. The postoperative training plan outlined here is not only based on this premise, but has been arranged specifically for use when the low friction Charnley prosthesis is employed.

## 1. IMMEDIATE POSTOPERATIVE CARE

When the patient's level of awareness permits, the therapist will encourage him to carry out the simple breathing exercises which have been previously taught; he will also encourage him to practise the foot and ankle movements designed to accelerate the venous return through the lower limbs.

Ward nursing staff have an important part to play in this form of care; from time to time they should remind the patient of the necessity of practising his exercises in the correct manner. This calls for close cooperation between nurse and therapist.

## 2. 1st AND 2nd POSTOPERATIVE DAYS

The therapist checks the position of the affected limb to ensure that the correct position of hip abduction has been maintained. It is also important to ensure that the hip is in a neutral position and has not fallen into lateral rotation. It should be noted that there is a marked tendency for the patient to move his trunk in line with the abducted limb. If this occurs the patient's trunk position must be adjusted so that he lies centrally in bed.

### Exercises

Quadriceps drill is started on the 1st postoperative day; usually this is confined to the sound limb. Contractions of the quadriceps of the affected limb are started when the vacuum drain is removed from the wound area (generally after 24 hours). It is important that the contractions are performed in a fairly slow and positive manner. Adequate periods of relaxation are essential.

With the surgeon's permission *gentle* flexion movements of the affected hip and knee are also started on the 1st postoperative day, the therapist giving maximum support. Assisted movement of this type should occupy only a brief period of time; in all, only about five careful flexion movements of hip and knee should be attempted. During this period of early hip movement the patient needs encouragement and reassurance.

In addition to this specific work, exercises to assist respiratory and circulatory function will be emphasized. (*See* Preoperative Exercise Programme, p. 223.)

Ideally, the therapist should arrange to visit the patient in the morning and afternoon for individual exercise sessions of about 10 minutes each.

## 3. FROM 2nd OR 3rd POSTOPERATIVE DAY UNTIL SUTURES ARE REMOVED BETWEEN 10th AND 14th DAY

### Standing, Walking and Sitting

Individual surgeons differ considerably with regard to the exact time when the patient is first allowed out of bed for standing and walking. Some allow this on the 2nd or 3rd postoperative day, while others postpone standing and walking for several days: this gives time for the patient to increase his range of hip flexion. It should be noted that some surgeons prefer their patients to be able to sit comfortably in a chair of suitable height before they attempt to stand and walk.

In the sitting position the patient must have his hips well abducted. Because of limited hip flexion many patients experience considerable difficulty in assuming a normal sitting position. To compensate for this the chair seat is 'angled' by the addition of two pillows, so that the patient assumes an inclined sitting position.

A stable well-designed armchair with the following features is an essential piece of equipment for an orthopaedic ward specializing in reconstructive hip surgery:

Adjustable legs, to ensure correct seat height;

Firm, non-sagging seat with cloth (rather than vinyl) covering;

High raked back, capable of easy adjustment;

Firm elongated arm rests to assist the patient in rising and lowering movements.

A Tubigrip bandage is often used on the affected leg to prevent oedema when the patient is ambulant or sitting in a chair. The bandage should extend from the webs of the toes to the tibial tubercle, and it is essential that the correct size of Tubigrip is used. It is also important that the support should be removed at night.

### Exercise Programme

Routine breathing, quadriceps, foot and ankle exercises are continued. Arm and shoulder girdle exercises are progressed in strength. Generally the patient is allowed to take a more normal half lying position.

Assisted active flexion of the hip and knee of the affected limb is continued as before, but the therapist encourages the patient to take a more active part.

The return movement of active extension is also emphasized. Some surgeons encourage assisted active abduction of the affected hip.

It is helpful if the patient spends short periods of time resting in the supine position. This not only assists in promoting a better posture but to some degree relieves the buttocks of pressure.

## 'Getting Up': The Initial Approach

For the majority of patients getting up for the first time after surgery and taking weight on the 'new' hip is something of a psychological ordeal, and they will need a considerable amount of reassurance from the therapist that all is well. It is most important that they should be given a clear idea of what is expected of them, and how they can be got on their feet safely without pain or discomfort.

Initially, the therapist will need a competent assistant to help in manœuvring the patient from the normal lying position to one in which he is positioned at right angles to the long axis of the bed. During this manœuvre it is essential for the affected limb to be fully supported by the therapist, and for the hips to be maintained in an abducted position. It is also important to prevent undue hip flexion.

During the main pivoting movement the patient will pull on the 'monkey' chain to relieve pressure on the buttocks; the assistant will support the trunk from the far side of the bed.

To bring the patient to the standing position he is next eased to the edge of the bed. When the buttocks are resting on the bed edge the therapist lowers the legs and at the same time the assistant helps to raise the patient's trunk. In this way the patient is manœuvred into the standing position with minimal hip flexion.

Throughout this movement the patient helps to minimize his body weight by the use of the 'monkey' chain.

*N.B.* Both the therapist and his assistant must be prepared to assist the patient immediately if he shows signs of fainting or distress due to the sudden change of body position.

### Using the Tilt Table

The use of a tilt table (either manually or electrically operated) simplifies the process of moving the patient from the horizontal to the vertical position, and is recommended.

Fundamentally, the tilt table consists of a padded platform which pivots on a stable tubular-steel base equipped with small braked wheels. The platform can be moved from the horizontal to the vertical position and can be stabilized effectively in any position between zero and 90°. The angle of inclination can be measured with the aid of the graduated angular scale incorporated in the table's design.

One end of the platform is equipped with a strong footrest; fold-away handles are provided on either side of the platform at about mid-position. Anchorage points are available for the use of restraining straps.

*Positioning the tilt table.* The tilt table is used in conjuction with a variable-height bed. The platform is set in a horizontal position alongside the bed (and securely braked) on the side of the patient's affected limb; the level of the platform and bed surface must be equal. The table is positioned as close to the bed edge as possible.

Before transferring the patient from the bed to the tilt table the platform surface should be covered with a sheet or cellular blanket. The covering not only adds to the patient's comfort but provides an easy means of adjusting his position when he is resting on the platform. Pillows are wedged longitudinally into the gap which exists between the edge of the platform and the bed.

*Transferring the patient.* In transferring the patient from the bed to the tilt table the therapist needs the help of two assistants. The therapist and one assistant kneel on the platform, facing the bed; the second assistant stands at the far side of the bed.

The patient (who lies in a supine position on the bed with his legs abducted) grasps the 'monkey' strap or chain, which is arranged on the overhead fixation point as near to the tilt table as possible so that its angle of inclination assists in the transference process. The patient's legs are well supported by the therapist; his seat and trunk are supported by the assistant kneeling alongside the therapist.

The patient is transferred by stages to the tilt table by the combined efforts of the kneeling supporters; their actions are reinforced by the patient using the 'monkey' strap or chain to take some of his body weight. The second assistant (who initially helped in the transference while standing by the bedside) now kneels on the bed to provide support and help in the final stage of the process. During this stage it is necessary for the kneeling supporters to move backwards into standing.

Once securely positioned on the platform of the tilt table, with a pillow under his head, the patient is eased carefully down the platform until the soles of his feet make firm contact with the footrest; the hips remain in an abducted position with the toes pointing upwards. The hand grips are positioned so that when the patient grasps them his elbows will be slightly flexed.

*Tilting the patient.* A very careful and *gradual* adjustment of the platform from the horizontal to the vertical position is then carried out. The actual time spent in reaching the vertical position can be extended, as thought necessary, by giving the patient short rest periods in various inclined positions. In this way the patient's circulatory system has time to adjust to the overall change of posture.

## Training in Standing and Walking

Initially the patient should stand with the help of a walking frame of a suitable height. He should be trained to stand in a good balanced position with his feet slightly apart. Once he has sufficient confidence to take weight evenly on both legs he is encouraged to carry out some simple exercises, e.g. hip and knee flexion of the affected leg through a comfortable range, followed by hip extension and abduction. Simple 'walking' movements are then carried out within the compass of the frame. This is very useful for boosting the patient's morale.

A brief period of walking with the assistance of the frame is used as a preliminary to walking with elbow crutches. Walking with crutches is best practised in a relatively small area; this gives the patient confidence and allows him to concentrate on his gait.

The patient should be taught to move both crutches forwards with the affected leg, and to take small even steps. Later on, a reciprocal walking pattern with the crutches is adopted. Care must be taken not to overdo walking training in the early stages, bearing in mind the patient's age and general condition.

The patient must be warned against making sudden changes of direction when walking; this can produce rotation stresses at the 'new' hip joint. Turning movements are best carried out by either describing a wide arc or using a series of small hitching movements of the pelvis (lateral tilting).

*Walking with sticks.* Some patients are able to progress rapidly to walking with two sticks, and are encouraged by their surgeons to do so. The majority of patients, however, use elbow crutches for a week or two after they have been discharged home. Much depends on the patient's general capability and home circumstances.

## 4. WHEN SUTURES HAVE BEEN REMOVED (10th–14th DAY) AND PATIENT REMAINS IN HOSPITAL FOR A DAY OR SO

The programme of ambulation and exercise is progressed. The distance covered in walking will be gradually increased and should include uneven areas and sloping surfaces. The technique of negotiating steps, stairs and curbs will be practised.

In association with the occupational therapist and the social worker the therapist should check on the patient's home circumstances in relation to his physical ability. It may be necessary for simple aids to daily living to be provided in the home, e.g. raised toilet seat, bath board, and suitable armchair of correct seat height.

Before being discharged from the ward the patient must be given advice on how to cope safely at home, with special reference to the avoidance of certain postures which put stress on the 'new' hip.

Adduction of the hips should be avoided, particularly in sitting and lying. When resting in bed on his sound side the patient should always have a firm pillow arranged longitudinally between the legs. Sitting on low chairs and settees, which emphasizes hip flexion, must also be avoided.

The patient should be instructed to keep his overall body weight within reasonable limits, so as to avoid overloading the prosthesis. He should also be advised to spend short periods of time (if feasible) in prone lying.

*Pool therapy.* Provided the wound area is soundly healed, and the surgeon approves, pool therapy can be used with considerable advantage to improve the function of the lower limbs and body as a whole. It also provides a pleasant variation of the exercise programme. Patients for pool therapy need to be selected with considerable care.

*Outpatient treatment.* It is helpful if the patient attends the hospital rehabilitation department two or three times a week for about 2–3 weeks after he has been discharged from the ward. This enables the therapist to check on his gait and general progress, and determine whether he needs one or two sticks in place of crutches. At this stage of recovery many patients do not require any form of walking aid.

## OTHER ASPECTS OF TOTAL HIP REPLACEMENT
## REVISION ARTHROPLASTY

In conditions where the original prosthesis has to be replaced due to mechanical failure or infection, the initial period of immobilization is extended considerably. It may consist of a 3-week period of complete bed rest. The treatment régime previously described (pp. 225–230) is then modified according to the surgeon's specific instructions.

## ARTHROPLASTY FOLLOWING JOINT DISEASE IN CHILDHOOD

When total hip replacement is used to restore movement in old joint conditions which have resulted in obliteration of the joint surfaces (bony ankylosis following acute suppurative arthritis or tuberculosis in childhood), both the initial period of immobilization and the treatment régime previously described are modified considerably, as indicated above.

After restoration of joint movement one of the most difficult problems facing both surgeon and therapist is the weakness of the controlling hip muscles. The original joint disease may have severely damaged, or obliterated, some of the main muscle groups. Considerable instability of the joint may occur.

## REFERENCES
Adams J. C. (1980) *Standard Orthopaedic Operations*, 2nd ed. Edinburgh, Churchill Livingstone.
Duthie R. B. and Ferguson A. B. (1973) *Mercer's Orthopaedic Surgery*, 7th ed. Edinburgh, Churchill Livingstone.

Edmonson A. S. and Crenshaw A. H. (ed.) (1980) *Campbell's Operative Orthopaedics*, Vol. 2, 6th ed. St Louis, Mosby, pp. 2319–2324.
Longton E. B. (1973) Orthopaedic surgery in arthritic lower-limb joints. *Physiotherapy* **59**, 116–119.
Longton E. B. (1982) Personal communication.

# 22. Meniscectomy

Meniscectomy is performed after an injury to a meniscus when the diagnosis of splitting and displacement is beyond doubt, e.g. when the meniscus has been displaced on more than one occasion.

## TYPES OF INCISION

### Excision of Medial Meniscus

Two main types of incision are used: the oblique incision and the transverse incision.

The *oblique incision*, 3·8–5 cm in length, begins close to the inframedial aspect of the patella and extends downwards and slightly backwards to a point about 1·2 cm below the joint line. The structures involved include skin, subcutaneous tissues, capsule, and synovial membrane of the knee joint.

The infrapatellar branch of the saphenous nerve may be divided. This causes temporary anaesthesia of the small zone of skin on the anterior aspect of the knee joint which is supplied by this nerve, and sometimes persistent tenderness of the scar. Smillie (1978a) states: 'The presence of the patellar plexus implies that sensory overlap is well developed in this region, and it is thus unusual for an area of diminished cutaneous sensation to remain permanently.'

The *traverse incision*, about 3·8 cm in length, is made over the anteromedial aspect of the knee joint, parallel with the articular surface of the tibia, and about 1·2 cm above it. This incision does not damage the infrapatellar nerve and provides good exposure. If the incision is placed too low the scar may become adherent to the surface of the tibia.

### Excision of Lateral Meniscus

The technique of approach is similar to that used for excision of the medial meniscus.

## ESSENTIALS OF TREATMENT

Orthopaedic surgeons differ with regard to the type of immobilization and management employed in the postoperative phase of treatment. Three régimes that are widely used are outlined here with the appropriate exercise therapy.

## 1. Non-weight-bearing Régime

After the operation the knee is immobilized by a firm flannel or domette-and-wool compression bandage; this helps to prevent postoperative haemarthrosis. The patient rests in bed for about two to three days until he has good quadriceps control and can perform straight leg raising satisfactorily. A pillow is sometimes used to support the limb; it is placed under the lower leg and does not extend to the knee joint. Its purpose is to maintain the straight position of the joint.

After about the 3rd postoperative day the patient is allowed out of bed for short periods of sitting and walking. When sitting the affected limb must be supported in a horizontal position by a stool and pillows or foam rubber gutter trough. Walking is restricted to a non-weight bearing technique with elbow crutches.

Non-weight-bearing is continued until the stitches are removed on the 10th or 12th postoperative day. During this phase the patient may be discharged home or remain in the ward.

After the stitches have been removed a crêpe bandage is applied to the knee joint to control oedema and provide some degree of support. The patient then makes a gradual progression from partial to full weight-bearing.

*Exercise Therapy*

Exercises to maintain the strength of the quadriceps femoris muscle are started on the 1st postoperative day. Generally the patient can contract the quadriceps statically, although in some cases it may be difficult to overcome the reflex inhibition of the muscle.

Transient pain localized to the site of the operation is to be expected on starting quadriceps exercises. It results from the drag on the incision produced by the contracting muscle.

AFTER REMOVAL OF SUTURES

The main aims consist of redeveloping the quadriceps femoris muscle, re-educating walking, and (if flexion exercises are allowed) restoring knee flexion. The reaction of the knee to weight-bearing and exercise must be observed very carefully; any marked increase of effusion indicates that the amount of activity allowed must be decreased and knee flexion omitted until the effusion has subsided.

The length of time required to achieve full recovery after a meniscectomy depends to a considerable extent on the patient's occupation. 'Experience has shown that whereas a clerk can return to his desk in the 4th week, a degree of physical fitness which will withstand the rigours of athletic activities is rarely possible in less than twelve weeks of organized rehabilitation. This applies in equal degree to those engaged in the manual occupations of heavy industry' (Smillie, 1978b).

ALLOWING KNEE FLEXION

Opinion varies among surgeons as to when knee flexion is to be allowed. Some consider that knee flexion exercises should not be used until the later phases of recovery, because in the earlier stages the movements may irritate the joint and produce an effusion. They stress that knee flexion usually returns by itself without any difficulty. Surgeons who hold this opinion will, in the absence of marked effusion, generally allow the patient to flex the knee within a pain-free range of movement once or twice daily about two weeks after the operation.

Other surgeons allow gentle knee flexion exercises between the 10th and 14th postoperative days, provided they are kept within a painless range of movement and there is no significant joint effusion.

## 2. Early Weight-bearing Régime (after 5 days)

Immediately after the operation the knee is immobilized in extension by a firm flannel or domette-and-wool compression bandage; this helps to prevent postoperative haemarthrosis. A gutter-type back splint is sometimes used in addition.

The patient rests in bed for approximately 5 days with the affected limb elevated (foam rubber trough resting either on pillows or on an adjustable elevation frame). After five days the back splint is discarded and, provided that straight leg raising can be performed satisfactorily, the patient is allowed out of bed for short periods of walking practice (partial weight-bearing with elbow crutches).

The stitches are removed between the 10th and 12th postoperative days, and the patient is discharged from the ward. A crêpe bandage is applied to the knee joint to control oedema and provide some degree of support. Full weight-bearing is allowed.

*Exercise Therapy*

As described previously (p. 233).

## 3. Early Weight-bearing Régime (with Plaster Cylinder)

After the operation a well-padded plaster cylinder is applied to the affected limb; it extends from the upper third of the thigh to just above the malleoli. During the application of the cylinder the lower edge is well padded with adhesive orthopaedic foam. This helps to maintain the position of the cylinder when the patient is in the erect position and prevents the lower edge from impinging on the dorsum of the foot. (Instead of a plaster cylinder some surgeons prefer to use a Raymed wrap-around back splint or 'knee immobilizer'.* The splint is applied over the compression bandage and extends from the upper third of the thigh to the ankle.

The patient rests in bed for about 2 days to allow the plaster to dry thoroughly and for quadriceps exercises—and, if possible, straight leg raising—to be practised. In general, the patient is allowed out of bed for short periods of standing and walking practice (partial weight-bearing with elbow crutches) on the 3rd postoperative day.

When the patient's walking and control of the affected limb are considered satisfactory he is allowed home. (It is important that he can negotiate stairs safely.) The plaster cylinder and stitches are usually removed between the 10th and 12th postoperative days, the patient returning to the hospital out-patients' department for these procedures.

A crêpe bandage is applied to the knee to control oedema and provide some degree of support. In general, partial weight-bearing with elbow crutches is continued for a few days until the patient has regained full control of the knee. The transition from partial to full weight-bearing without elbow crutches must be gradual. Much will depend on the individual's reaction to pain and whether the joint is free of effusion.

*Exercise Therapy*
As described previously (p. 233).

## MENISCECTOMY WITH COMPLICATIONS

Severe pain and reactionary effusion of the knee are associated with certain complications which may arise during or after the operation. Such complications include: (1) Trauma during the operation, and (2) Postoperative haemarthrosis.

Of trauma at operation Smillie (1978c) states: ' . . . Cases in which the operation is performed only with difficulty and in which the medial ligament and capsule are subjected to prolonged stretching . . . and the synovial membrane exposed to prolonged pressure . . . frequently suffer from persistent synovitis. . . .' Postoperative haemarthrosis may occur as a result of inadequate compression of the knee by the bandage or padding of the plaster

---

* The 'knee immobilizer' consists of a tapered back splint incorporating 4 removable metal struts, one each on the lateral and medial aspects and 2 on the posterior aspect. It is constructed from fabric-backed felt with a Velcro 'fold-back' closure system which allows a degree of adjustability. The 'immobilizer' is obtainable from Raymed (a division of Charles F. Thackray Ltd.), of Viaduct Road, Leeds, LS4 2BR.

cylinder. The condition gives rise to adhesions, residual synovial thickenings, and persistent effusion.

Patients with a marked reaction of the knee will experience increased pain when they attempt to exercise the quadriceps femoris muscle. The authors are of the opinion that patients should not be bullied into exercising the muscle (as is often done), but allowed to rest the limb until the main reaction of the joint has subsided and a static contraction of the quadriceps can be obtained without difficulty. (This does not mean, however, that the patient is allowed to forget his role in attempting to activate the quadriceps muscle.) Straight leg raising will usually be possible about a day later.

## EXERCISE THERAPY

The lists of exercises given here are intended to be a guide to the postoperative treatment of meniscectomy when any one of the three treatment régimes described (pp. 233–235) are used.

## PROGRAMME A: FOR USE WHEN KNEE IS IMMOBILIZED BY COMPRESSION BANDAGE, WITH OR WITHOUT A BACK SPLINT (Régimes 1 and 2, pp. 233–234.)

TABLE 1

From 1st postoperative day until straight leg raising can be performed without assistance: usually by 2nd or 3rd postoperative day.

*Remedial Aims*

PRIMARY
To maintain the quadriceps femoris muscle.

SECONDARY
1. To maintain the mobility of the toes, ankle, midtarsal and subtalar joints.
2. To maintain the muscles of the lower leg and hip joint.

*Exercise Period*
10 minutes, twice daily.

*N.B.* The patient must be instructed to contract the quadriceps femoris muscle *correctly* at least six times every half hour—'Give it six of the best . . .'.

**Primary Exercises**

*Quadriceps Exercises*

1. Half lying; single Quadriceps contractions.
2. Half lying (affected limb well supported by therapist: hip flexed to about 60°); 'holding' the position for a brief period.
3. As above; single Leg lowering with assistance.
4. Half crook side-lying (firm pillows supporting affected limb); single (affected) Knee bracing, followed by slight Leg raising sideways and carrying forwards. Initially, therapist provides support.
5. Half crook side-lying (firm pillows supporting affected limb); single (affected) Knee bracing, followed by slight Leg raising and carrying backwards. Initially, therapist provides support.

**Secondary Exercises**

*Lower Leg Exercises*

1. Half lying; Toe bending and stretching: both feet.
2. Half lying; (*a*) alternate Ankle bending and stretching, (*b*) alternate Foot turning inwards and outwards.
3. Half lying; (*a*) single Ankle bending, (*b*) single Ankle stretching.
4. Half lying; (*a*) single Foot turning inwards, (*b*) single Foot turning outwards.

*Hip Exercises*

5. Lying; single Gluteal contractions.
6. Lying; single and double Gluteal contractions.
7. Lying; single Leg downpressing.

TABLE 2

From 2nd or 3rd postoperative day until the 10th day (when stitches are removed).

The patient performs the exercises on the bed. Patients on the *non-weight-bearing régime* are allowed out of bed for short periods of sitting and walking (non-weight-bearing) from about the 3rd postoperative day.

Patients on the *weight-bearing régime* remain in bed for about 5 days after operation. Usually they are allowed out of bed on the 5th day for sitting, standing and walking (partial weight-bearing), provided they have control over the quadriceps muscle and can perform straight leg raising satisfactorily.

*Remedial Aims*

As in previous section.

*Exercise Period*

15–20 minutes, twice daily.

*N.B.* The patient must be instructed to contract the quadriceps femoris muscle *correctly* at least six times every half hour—'Give it six of the best . . .'.

## Primary Exercises

*Quadriceps Exercises*

1. Half lying; single and double Quadriceps contractions.
2. Half lying; combined (single) Quadriceps and Gluteal contractions.
3. Lying; single Leg downpressing.
4. Lying; single Leg raising. When the patient can perform straight leg raising without any difficulty weight resistance is added, with the surgeon's permission. Usually a weight of 0.5 kg is used at first. It is progressed gradually. The exercise must not be allowed to cause pain or to overfatigue the quadriceps muscle. Throughout the leg lifting and lowering the knee must be kept firmly braced.

## Secondary Exercises

*Lower Leg Exercises*

1. Half lying; (*a*) alternate Ankle bending and stretching, (*b*) alternate Foot turning inwards and outwards.
2. Half lying; single or double Foot circling.
3. Half lying; (*a*) single and double Ankle bending, (*b*) single and double Ankle stretching, (*c*) single and double Foot turning inwards.

*Hip Exercises*

4. Half crook side-lying; single (affected) slight Leg raising sideways, and carrying forwards and backwards to 6 counts. (*See Fig.* 189, p. 159.)
5. Half crook side-lying; single (affected) Leg raising sideways.
6. Forehead rest prone lying; single Knee bracing, followed by slight Leg raising backwards.

## PROGRAMME B: FOR USE WHEN KNEE IS IMMOBILIZED BY PLASTER CYLINDER OR RAYMED 'KNEE IMMOBILIZER'

TABLE OF EXERCISES

For first 2–3 postoperative days.

The patient rests in bed for about 2 days to allow the plaster to dry out. A plastic sheet is usually in position under the affected limb to protect the bedclothes. A bed cradle allows air circulation and prevents bedclothes from coming into contact with the damp plaster cast.

*N.B.* Before the patient starts his exercise programme the therapist should inspect the state of the entire plaster cylinder to ascertain if the plaster is intact; fine cracks can easily go undetected.

*Remedial Aims*

PRIMARY
To maintain the quadriceps femoris muscle.

SECONDARY
1. To maintain the mobility of the toes, ankle, midtarsal and subtalar joints.
2. To maintain the muscles of the lower leg and hip joint.

*Exercise Period*
10 minutes, twice daily.
   *N.B.* The patient must be instructed to contract the quadriceps femoris muscle *correctly* at least six times every half hour—'Give it six of the best . . .'.

## Primary Exercises

*Quadriceps Exercises*
1. Half lying; single Quadriceps contractions.
2. Half lying; single Knee bracing, followed by Hip turning inwards and outwards.
3. Lying; single Leg lifting (assistance from therapist) through 10–15°.
4. Half lying; single Knee bracing, followed by small range Hip abduction and adduction.

## Secondary Exercises

*Lower Leg Exercises*
1. Half lying; Toe bending and stretching: both feet.
2. Half lying; (*a*) alternate Ankle bending and stretching, (*b*) alternate Foot turning inwards and outwards.
3. Half lying; (*a*) single Ankle bending, (*b*) single Ankle stretching.
4. Half lying; (*a*) single Foot turning inwards, (*b*) single Foot turning outwards.

*Hip Exercises*
5. Lying; single Gluteal contractions.
6. Lying; single Leg downpressing.

**Progression of Exercise Programme**

On the 2nd or 3rd postoperative day the patient is allowed out of bed and is given instruction in standing and walking techniques. Elbow crutches are used for walking practice, and initially the patient is partial weight-bearing.

As a preliminary to walking training the patient practises hip strengthening exercises in the standing position: he can stabilize himself by holding on to the back of a suitable chair. Later he can carry out the movements while stabilized by the crutches. Hip updrawing movements (with knee firmly braced) are of particular value.

The patient is discharged home about the 4th postoperative day. It is most important that before he leaves the ward he has received adequate training in stair climbing with the help of crutches.

*N.B.* The patient must be aware of the importance of practising his exercises at home in the correct manner.

**PROGRAMME C: FOR USE AFTER 10th OR 12th POSTOPERATIVE DAY. THE EXERCISE TABLES HAVE BEEN ARRANGED TO SUIT THE REQUIREMENTS OF ANY OF THE THREE TREATMENT RÉGIMES DESCRIBED** (pp. 233–235)

TABLE 3

From 10th or 12th postoperative day, when stitches are removed, for about 2 weeks. Full weight-bearing is allowed. (If a non-weight-bearing régime has been followed previously, progression from partial to full weight-bearing must be gradual.) A crêpe bandage is worn on the knee to control oedema and to provide some support.

*Remedial Aims*

PRIMARY
1. To redevelop the quadriceps femoris muscle.
2. To restore the mobility of the knee joint.
3. To re-educate walking.

SECONDARY
1. To redevelop the muscles of the hip joint.
2. To re-educate neuromuscular co-ordination.

*Exercise Period*

30 minutes, once or twice daily. Additional time is required for the straight leg raising exercise against weight resistance.

## Primary Exercises

*Quadriceps Exercises*

1. Long sitting (trunk inclined backwards with hand support); single and double Quadriceps contractions.
2. Half lying or lying; single straight Leg raising against weight resistance.
3. Half lying or lying (wedge or pillow under affected knee); short range extension of knee, with or without weight resistance.*
4. High sitting (plinth: knees flexed comfortably to about 30°, with heels supported on stool); single Knee stretching.*

*Knee Flexion Exercises*

5. Lying; single Knee raising with heel kept in contact with supporting surface.*
6. Forehead rest prone lying; alternate Knee bending and stretching.*

*Walking*

7. Re-education in walking.

*N.B.* When the wound is fully healed and no effusion of the joint is present exercises in the pool may be used as an adjunct to the specific exercises suggested.

## TABLE 4

For use about a month after the operation. Some of the exercises suggested could be included as part of a Specific Exercise Circuit (p. 249).

*Remedial Aims*

PRIMARY

1. To redevelop the quadriceps femoris muscle.
2. To restore the mobility of the knee joint.

SECONDARY

1. To redevelop the extensor muscles of the hip joint.
2. To develop neuromuscular co-ordination.

*Exercise Period*

30 minutes, once daily. Additional time is required for the resisted knee extension exercise and graduated pool therapy.

---

* Not to be used in the presence of marked effusion of the knee, or if the surgeon does not permit knee flexion exercises (p. 234).

**Primary Exercises**

*Quadriceps Exercises*

1. Half wing half low yard grasp standing (wall bars); Heel raising and Knee bending.
2. Low reach grasp stride standing (wall bars); Heel raising and single Knee bending. (*See Fig.* 196, p. 165.)
3. Low reach grasp instep support standing (wall bars and stool); single Heel raising and Knee bending.
4. Skipping: (*a*) Skip jumps with a rebound, (*b*) High skip jumps.
5. High sitting (bench); single (affected) Knee stretching against weight or weight-and-pulley resistance.

*Knee Flexion Exercises*

6. Bend grasp high standing (wall bars); Knee bending and stretching with Hand travelling down and up the bars. (*See Fig.* 206, p. 169.)
7. Lying; cycling.

**Secondary Exercises**

*Balance Exercises*

1. Balance half standing (balance bench rib); balance walking fowards and backwards.
2. Balance walking with Knee and Arm raising of the same side, and opposite Arm raising backwards.
3. Toe balance walking along a straight line to 3 counts, followed by Knee full bending and stretching with the knees forwards to 6 counts.

*Hip Exercises*

4. Primary Exercises 1–4.

TABLE 5*

A final exercise programme suitable for use when a high degree of physical fitness is required.

*Remedial Aims*

As in previous section.

---

* Progressive circuit training with weight resistance forms a very useful alternative to the exercise table. So also does a pre-work circuit designed to simulate normal working stresses (*see* p. 251).

*Exercise Period*
As in previous section.

**Primary Exercises**

*Quadriceps Exercises*

1. Wing standing; Heel raising and Knee bending.
2. Wing stride standing; Heel raising and single Knee bending.
3. Wing instep support standing (stool); single Heel raising and Knee bending. (*See Fig.* 188, p. 157.)
4. Skipping: Hopping with a rebound and alternate Knee stretching. (*See Fig.* 8, p. 12.)
5. Bend standing; hopping with alternate Toe placing forwards (and opposite Arm stretching forwards), and alternate Toe placing sideways (with opposite Arm stretching sideways). (*See Fig.* 7, p. 12.)
6. Hopping with a rebound and opposite Knee and Arm raising.
7. Wing standing; hopping with a rebound and alternate Leg swinging sideways.
8. High sitting (bench); single (affected) Knee stretching against weight or weight-and-pulley resistance.

*Knee Flexion Exercise*

9. Forearm reach grasp kneeling (wall bars); attempting to assume kneel sitting. (*See Fig.* 208, p. 170.)

**Secondary Exercises**

*Balance Exercises*

1. Balance half standing (balance bench rib); balance walking forwards with Knee and Arm raising of the same side and opposite Arm raising backwards.
2. Balance half standing (balance bench rib); Toe balance walking forwards to 3 counts, followed by Knee full bending and stretching with knees forward to 6 counts.

*Hip Exercises*

3. Primary Exercises 1–7; Secondary Exercise 2.

**REFERENCES**
Smillie I. S. (1978a) *Injuries of the Knee Joint*, 5th ed. Edinburgh, Churchill Livingstone, p. 181.
Smillie I. S. (1978b) *Ibid.* p. 173.
Smillie I. S. (1978c) *Ibid.* p. 179.

# PART 5

# GENERAL EXERCISE THERAPY

In the broad sense general exercise therapy encompasses a wide spectrum of physical activity, ranging from informal movement and recreational pursuits to more organized and purposeful forms of exercise.

This section of the book deals with two widely differing aspects of general exercise in use today: progressive circuit training (representing an intensive and highly organized form of movement) and exercises to music, which represent a more informal approach to general exercise.

# 23. Progressive circuit training

Circuit training was originally evolved by Morgan and Adamson in the early 1950s, and was designed as a system of exercise training for maintaining and increasing physical fitness. It is capable of being adapted for all ability levels and aims at progressively developing endurance, strength, function and cardio-respiratory efficiency.

Fundamentally, circuit training consists of a number of performers carrying out a series of pre-determined exercises, with or without apparatus, which are arranged in a definite sequence. The floor areas in which the activities are performed are known as 'exercise' or 'task stations'. The stations are visited in turn by the performers and the movements indicated for each individual are performed against a prescribed time allocation.

Three circuit laps are completed with increasing rapidity, each successive lap taking less time than the previous one. During the final circuit lap the performers are working at maximum capacity. Several variations of this theme are possible (p. 254).

It should be noted that a circuit may be the main core of a specific exercise session, or the culmination of a general fitness programme.


## TYPES OF CIRCUIT

There are four distinct types of circuit: (1) *General Circuit* (*Fig.* 222*a*), which aims at providing an overall fitness programme (p. 248); (2) *Specific Circuit* (*Fig.* 222*b*), which is used to exercise a particular body region with special reference to strengthening and mobilizing (p. 249); (3) *Function Circuit* (*Fig.* 222*c*), which utilizes the types of movement encountered in ordinary daily living as distinct from gymnastic exercises (p. 250); and (4) *Pre-work Circuit* (*Fig.* 222*d*), which provides a series of realistic work situations with emphasis on manual skills (p. 251).


## PRACTICAL APPLICATION

In a full circuit there are normally 7 or 8 exercise stations. The performer works at each exercise task for a set period of time, usually 1 minute. He

# General Fitness Circuits for 7 Exercises

## These indicate how a theme may be modified to promote interest, and progress physical output.

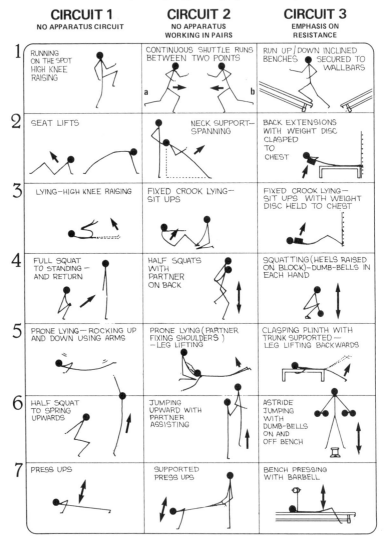

| CIRCUIT 1 | CIRCUIT 2 | CIRCUIT 3 |
|---|---|---|
| NO APPARATUS CIRCUIT | NO APPARATUS WORKING IN PAIRS | EMPHASIS ON RESISTANCE |
| 1 RUNNING ON THE SPOT HIGH KNEE RAISING | CONTINUOUS SHUTTLE RUNS BETWEEN TWO POINTS | RUN UP/DOWN INCLINED BENCHES SECURED TO WALLBARS |
| 2 SEAT LIFTS | NECK SUPPORT— SPANNING | BACK EXTENSIONS WITH WEIGHT DISC CLASPED TO CHEST |
| 3 LYING—HIGH KNEE RAISING | FIXED CROOK LYING— SIT UPS | FIXED CROOK LYING— SIT UPS WITH WEIGHT DISC HELD TO CHEST |
| 4 FULL SQUAT TO STANDING— AND RETURN | HALF SQUATS WITH PARTNER ON BACK | SQUATTING (HEELS RAISED ON BLOCK)—DUMB-BELLS IN EACH HAND |
| 5 PRONE LYING—ROCKING UP AND DOWN USING ARMS | PRONE LYING (PARTNER FIXING SHOULDERS) —LEG LIFTING | CLASPING PLINTH WITH TRUNK SUPPORTED— LEG LIFTING BACKWARDS |
| 6 HALF SQUAT TO SPRING UPWARDS | JUMPING UPWARD WITH PARTNER ASSISTING | ASTRIDE JUMPING WITH DUMB-BELLS ON AND OFF BENCH |
| 7 PRESS UPS | SUPPORTED PRESS UPS | BENCH PRESSING WITH BARBELL |

*Fig.* 222a. General Fitness Circuit.

# Specific Leg Circuit

**AIMS:** To redevelop quadriceps femoris muscle, to restore mobility of hip and knee, and to improve general fitness.

| | DESCRIPTION | TASK | SCORING |
|---|---|---|---|
| 1 | RIDE SITTING (BALANCE BENCH: BUTTOCKS ON FOLDED TOWEL) — FORWARD AND BACKWARD PROPULSION OF BODY BY LEGS | 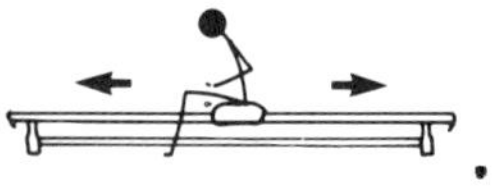 | TOTAL EACH LENGTH COMPLETED |
| 2 | FIXED LYING (PILLOW UNDER BUTTOCKS) — SIT UPS | 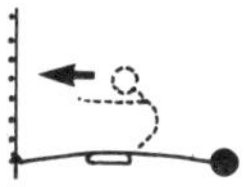 | COUNT EACH SIT UP |
| 3 | STANDING (HANDS GRASPING ONE END OF INCLINED BALANCE BENCH) — SQUATTING WITH FEET FLAT ON FLOOR | 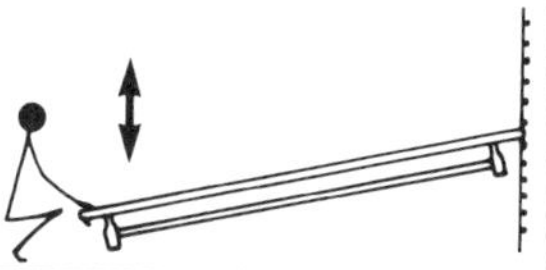 | TOTAL EACH SQUAT |
| 4 | INCLINED PRONE FALLING — 'WALKING' LEGS FORWARD AND BACKWARD | 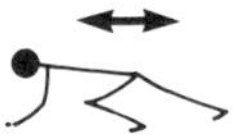 | TOTAL EACH LEG MOVEMENT |
| 5 | DUCKING UNDER LOW ROPE TO STAND UPRIGHT: CONTINUOUS FLOW | 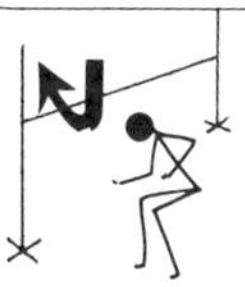 | COUNT EACH DUCK UNDER ROPE |
| 6 | STEP UPS (STOOL OR BALANCE BENCH) WITH DUMBELLS — AFFECTED LEG LEADING | 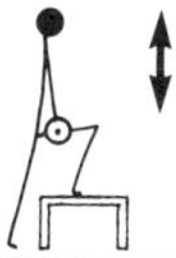 | TOTAL EACH STEP UP |
| 7 | ALTERNATE SEAT AND LEG RAISING TO ROLL MEDICINE BALL ALONG LEGS | 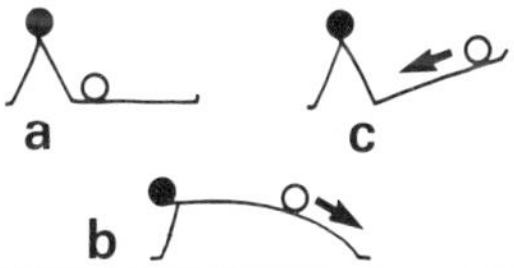 | COUNT EACH SUCCESSFUL ROLL OF BALL |

*Fig. 222b.* Specific Leg Circuit.

# Function Circuit

**The circuit is designed to reinforce the functional skills that may be required at home. The activities are performed at a steady pace.**

| | DESCRIPTION | TASK | SCORING |
|---|---|---|---|
| 1 | SITTING AND RISING— MOVING FROM STOOL TO STOOL | 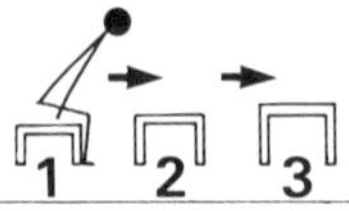 | COUNT NUMBER OF STOOL CHANGES |
| 2 | CRAWLING ON ALL FOURS OVER OBSTACLE TO STAND AT WALL BARS— AND RETURN | 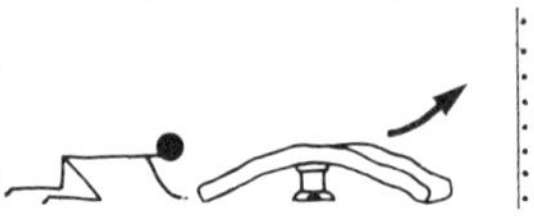 | COUNT EACH LAP |
| 3 | ROLLING FROM PRONE TO SUPINE LYING | 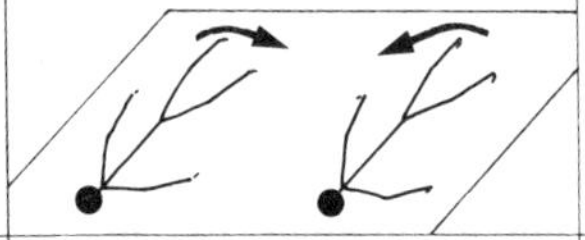 | COUNT POSITION CHANGES |
| 4 | PUSHING LOADED WHEELCHAIR OR TROLLEY OVER MEASURED DISTANCE OR AROUND OBSTACLES | 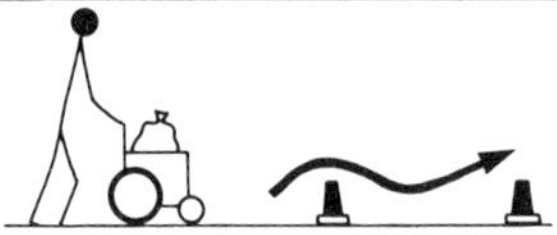 | TOTAL OBSTACLES NEGOTIATED, HIT, OR DISTANCE TRAVELLED |
| 5 | STAIR CLIMBING ON SEAT WITH BACK TO STAIRS— AND RETURN IN SAME POSITION | 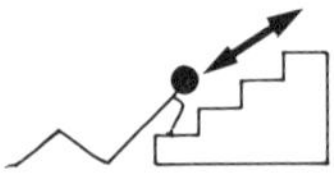 | COUNT EACH SINGLE STAIR NEGOTIATED |
| 6 | PICKING UP BEAN BAGS FROM FLOOR TO PLACE IN BUCKET SUSPENDED AT HEAD HEIGHT | 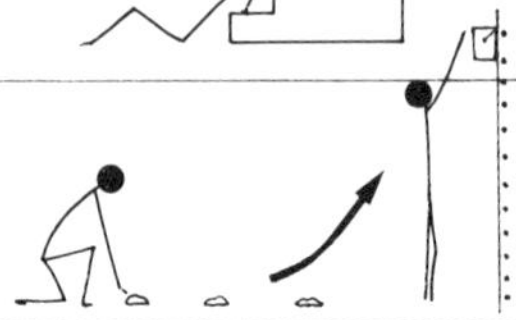 | TOTAL BEAN BAGS IN BUCKET |
| 7 | WALKING WITH CARE OVER RUBBER MATS OR UNEVEN SOFT SURFACES | 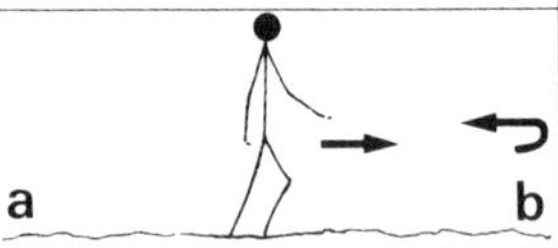 | ADD LAPS OR DISTANCE TRAVELLED |
| 8 | STEPPING UP AND DOWN ON FIRST STEP (BANISTER AND STICK SUPPORT IF NECESSARY) | 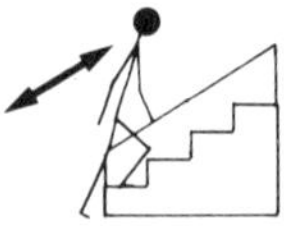 | COUNT EACH TIME BOTH FEET ARE TOGETHER, OR SINGLE STEPS |

*Fig.* 222c. Function Circuit.

# Pre-work Circuit

**N.B. It is important to indicate and mark clearly weight of articles to be lifted.**

| | DESCRIPTION | TASK | SCORE |
|---|---|---|---|
| 1 | SHOVELLING RUBBER MEDICINE BALLS INTO AREA 'A', THEN BACK INTO AREA 'B' — QUICKLY | 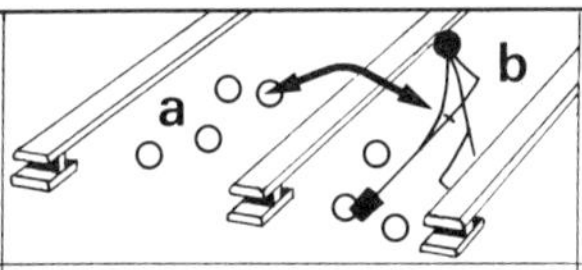 | COUNT BALLS SHOVELLED |
| 2 | PUSHING LOW, LOADED TROLLEY BETWEEN TWO POINTS — AND TURNING | 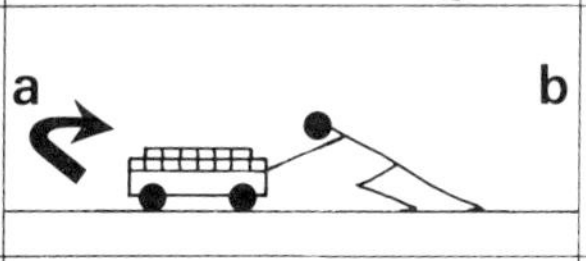 | TOTAL LAPS |
| 3 | STACKING MILK CRATES FILLED WITH BRICKS TO CHEST HEIGHT FROM 'A' TO 'B' THEN 'B' TO 'A' | 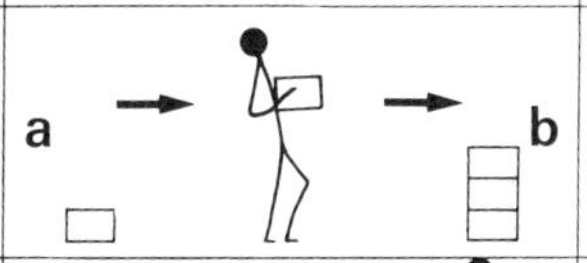 | TOTAL CRATES STACKED |
| 4 | CLIMBING UP WELL SECURED LADDER — AND RETURN | 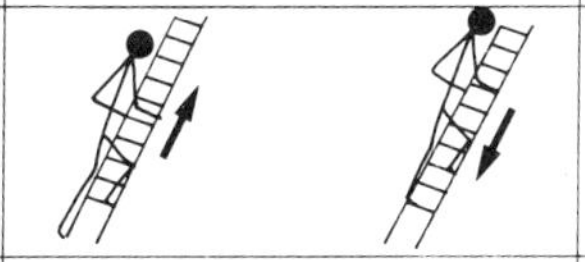 | COUNT ASCENDS AND DESCENDS |
| 5 | LIFTING PIT PROP OR LONG LOG FROM FLOOR TO SHOULDER-SURMOUNTING OBSTACLES-AND RETURN | 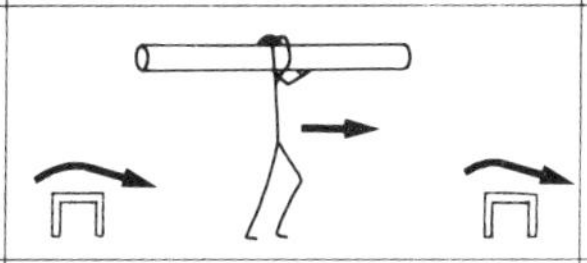 | TOTAL LAPS OR DISTANCE TRAVELLED |
| 6 | ROLLING UNDER 1ST HURDLE, CRAWLING UNDER 2ND, STEPPING OVER 3RD, AND CLIMBING THROUGH 4TH | 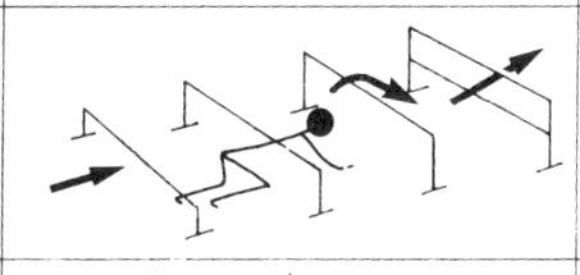 | COUNT HAZARDS COMPLETED |
| 7 | CARRY LARGE REINFORCED BAG OF LINEN FROM 'A' TO 'B', LOWER TO FLOOR, AND DRAG BACKWARDS FROM 'B' TO 'A' | 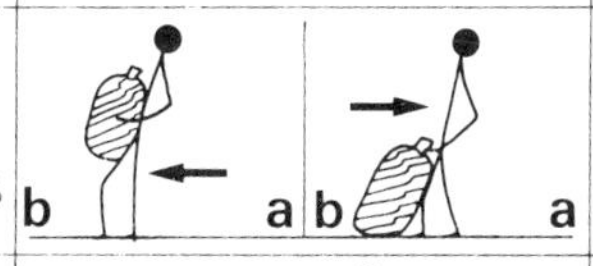 | COUNT LIFTS AND DRAGS |
| 8 | ROLLING OIL DRUM OR BARREL, FILLED WITH SAND, UP SLIGHT INCLINE — THEN DOWN AND RETURN | 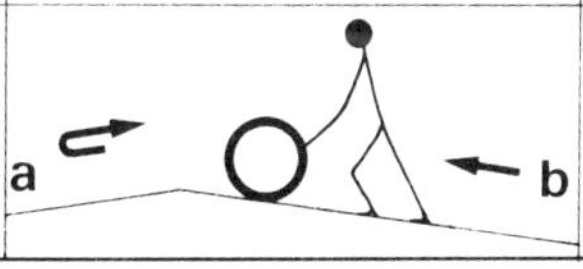 | TOTAL UPS AND DOWNS |

*Fig.* 222d. Pre-work Circuit.

works as quickly as possible and then moves on to another exercise station. In this way he completes all the set work for the full circuit of exercises.

At the end of the first circuit lap the performer has a short rest. The second and third circuit laps are performed in a similar manner to the first. At the third and final lap the performer is working at maximum capacity.

*Fixing the Repetition Dose.* The repetition level or dose of each exercise in the circuit must be established for each performer. A useful method of fixing the dose is to time the maximum number of repetitions achieved by the performer at each activity over a period of 1 minute (with only brief rest intervals being allowed between the various activities). The scores recorded in this way are halved and these become the performer's training doses.

The performer's time for three laps at his training doses or levels is recorded. He aims at attempting to reduce this time before re-testing takes place.

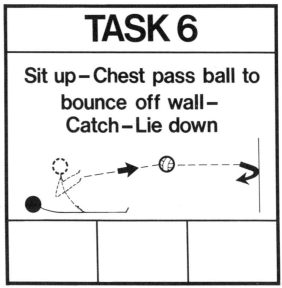

*Fig.* 223. A numbered circuit guide board. The boards are placed alongside the activity stations and are used to record the scores for individual circuit tasks.

*Scoring.* The score for individual circuit tasks can be recorded on the circuit guide boards (*Fig.* 223). A number of different methods of scoring is used. Some examples are given here.

1. Count the number of repetitions performed at an individual task in a set time. Then, taking the lap as a whole, total up all the repetitions performed. This procedure is followed for the three laps.

2. Allocate a set number of repetitions at each exercise station. Check the time taken to complete the activity. When the first circuit is completed total up all the times. This procedure is followed for the three laps.

3. If the performer has a task involving moving over a distance it can be recorded in (a) time taken to complete distance, (b) actual distance covered and measured, and (c) number of laps completed between the two set points.

4. When a pair of performers work at some tasks separately, individual score totals may be added together. If sharing one task the same procedure is followed. This method of scoring can also be used when a team of performers work together at a circuit.

5. If a skill element is included in the circuit the score can be considered from the viewpoint of movement or time. For example, in basketball shooting the number of baskets scored in a set time can be recorded, or the time it takes to score a number of baskets.

## SETTING STANDARDS

Circuit activities must be carefully selected and graduated, so that they are well within the physical capabilities of the performers; unfortunately, this is sometimes overlooked.

The individual tasks vary considerably, depending on the degree of mental and physical effort required. In evaluating the performers' repetition levels the instructor must perform the activities himself, so that he can accurately gauge the individual and cumulative effort required.

In organizing circuits for a group of performers with varying standards of physical ability a simple three-tier grading system, associated with distinctive colours, is sometimes used, e.g. White Circuit (simple activities), Blue Circuit (more advanced tasks), and Red Circuit (the most strenuous activities). This colour coding is carried through to the circuit boards, where any reference to a particular circuit is given in the appropriate colour. This makes for easy recognition of the various modifications to be undertaken by individual performers.

Circuit training in any form makes strong physical demands on the performer. Before taking part it is essential to 'warm up' thoroughly. On completion of a strenuous circuit a short period should be spent in relaxed walking or gentle jogging on the spot. This provides a suitable 'run down' after effort.

## METHOD OF TIMING CIRCUIT

Accurate timing of a circuit can be achieved by the use of a stopwatch held by the instructor. Alternatively, a large-faced clock with second sweep hand (positioned so that it can be seen easily by the performers) can be used.

Timing is best registered by a battery of three Smith-type lever-operated timing clocks, mounted on a wooden base and protected by a metal carrying handle (*Fig.* 224). Two of the clocks are second-elapsed timers; they are used individually to time two separate performers. The third clock (a second-interval timer) is used for overall timing.

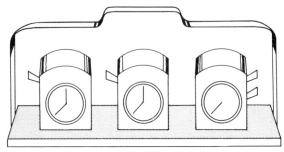

*Fig.* 224. Timing is best registered by a battery of three lever-operated timing clocks. Two of the clocks are second-elapsed timers. The third clock is a second-interval timer.

It is a useful practice for the instructor to indicate verbally the progress of time at intervals while the circuit is being worked. When the speed of the activity is relatively slow, repetition counting can be done by the performers. If the pace is fast and demanding, however, it is best for a non-performer to carry out this function.

## INTRODUCING THE CIRCUIT

When a circuit has been devised and levels of performance set, the performers should try out the exercise tasks in their own time. This, coupled with good coaching, should develop correct technique of performance—*not* to be lost when working under pressure.

A numbered circuit guide board (*Fig.* 223), painted matt black with simple diagrams and exercise instructions, is placed alongside each activity station. The direction taken by the performers round the circuit can be indicated by a series of large arrows chalked on the floor.

After a session of circuit training it is extremely useful to encourage the performers to give their opinion on the effectiveness of the lay-out and range of activities used.

## VARIATIONS OF CIRCUIT TRAINING

Some of the most useful practical variations include:
  1. Rearranging the circuit tasks in a different order.

2. Allowing the circuit tasks to be selected by the performers in order of preference.

3. Changing the starting positions of some of the exercises, e.g. substituting Press Ups for Bench Pressing.

4. Varying the apparatus while maintaining the same effect, e.g. using Leg Press machine in place of Squats with Weights.

5. Allowing the timing of the circuit to be one of the tasks: this gives a rest period to each of the performers.

6. Arranging for the performers to work in pairs. One counts the repetitions while the other works: the roles are then reversed.

7. Beat the score. On concluding a task the performer chalks the score achieved on the floor and initials it. The next performer who attempts the task endeavours to exceed this score, and so on.

8. Splitting the circuit into two sections and the performers into two groups—work each section separately and then change.

9. Adding a skill task, such as basketball shooting: points are included for scoring.

## EQUIPMENT

Most conventional gymnastic equipment can be used for circuit training: wall bars, climbing frames, balance benches, parallel bars, stools, climbing ropes and mats. Weight resistance apparatus is also used: barbells, dumb-bells, calf-machines, squat stands and leg press machines. The all-purpose 'multi-gym' (which includes a selection of weight training equipment) is also extremely useful.

Small equipment can be usefully employed: medicine balls of different weights, basketballs, footballs, bean bags, hoops and ash poles.

A wide selection of equipment for functional circuits is required: wooden crates, barrels, oil drums, scaffolding and planking, wheelbarrows, tyres of different sizes, ladders, chains, bricks and shovels.

## CLOTHING

The type of clothing required will depend on the nature of the circuit employed. Strenuous work needs the minimum of clothing: sleeveless T-shirts, shorts and gym shoes. Functional activities are best carried out with protection for knees and elbows, and a light track suit is recommended. Ideally, pre-work activities need to be performed in the protective clothing of the particular occupation simulated.

## REFERENCE

Morgan R. E. and Adamson G. T. (1961) *Circuit Training*, 2nd ed. London, Bell.

# 24. Exercises to music

In many rehabilitation centres and health clubs morning and afternoon treatment sessions start with a 20–30 minute period of 'warming-up' exercises to music. This provides a lively start to the sessions and presents general exercises in a stimulating and acceptable form.

In hospital practice there is rarely time to give properly organized periods of general exercises and this aspect of treatment tends to be neglected. The difficulty can be overcome to some extent by arranging a 5 or 6 minute period of general 'warming-up' exercises to recorded music before the specific exercise period.

## STARTING POSITIONS

In general, standing and sitting are the best starting positions to use for 'warming-up' exercises; they allow patients to observe the instructor without difficulty. The lying position can be used but coaching and change of exercise are made more difficult.

In organizing a class of patients with mixed disabilities it is best for the more able patients to stand and the more disabled to exercise in sitting. The leader, facing the class, performs the movements in time to the music and the class follows his lead. Ideally, there should be no break between individual exercises, and the movements should flow as naturally as possible into each other.

To provide an overall balance of activity, and prevent undue fatigue, the instructor should not dwell too long on any one exercise.

## SEQUENCE OF EXERCISES

The warming-up programme is arranged in such a way that all parts of the body are exercised in turn. To achieve variety of movement and avoid fatigue of any one muscle group it is helpful to start with the upper aspect of the body and progress downwards, and then repeat this sequence with different exercises, as indicated in the specimen tables (p. 258).

## STEREO EQUIPMENT AND MUSIC

Essential equipment consists of a good, well-sprung record deck capable of taking long and single play records, plus amplifier and two speaker units.

For normal class work the volume output should be set at a reasonable level with the bass volume gently obvious. It should be possible for class members to hear the leader's instructions without difficulty.

It is not easy to select music which is acceptable to the individual taste of the various class members and which at the same time matches the character of the movements. To overcome this problem a wide selection of music is used, ranging from classical to 'pop', and including synthesized music. Both instrumental and vocal recordings are used.

## MUSIC FOR MOVEMENT

No attempt has been made to list individual records, with their serial numbers, of particular types of music. Popular records have a relatively short life and quickly become unobtainable. It has been considered more useful to suggest the names of individual band leaders and groups whose music or interpretations have been found of value in matching music to movement.

Recordings made by the following artistes are extremely useful: Herb Alpert and his Tijuana Brass, Bert Kaempfert and his Orchestra, Geoff Love and his Orchestra, Kenny Ball and his Jazzmen, and James Last and his Orchestra.

Certain piano pieces played in strict tempo are also of value, e.g. interpretations by Charlie Kunz and recordings of Scott Joplin's works.

## WIDENING INTEREST

Simple equipment, such as sticks, balls, hoops and dumb-bells, can be used to great advantage in widening the interest and scope of some of the activities which form the exercise tables. Equipment of this sort also lends itself to partner activities performed in time to the music. For example, (a) partners facing in walk forwards standing, and grasping ends of sticks, alternate Arm moving backwards and forwards (rhythmical 'piston' action), and (b) ball bouncing between partners facing each other.

Singing while moving to music is another way of increasing the patients' participation in the exercise programme. This can occur spontaneously; on other occasions it is initiated by the instructor. At all times it is essential to keep this form of expression under control. If overdone, singing can easily disrupt the class and undermine the authority of the instructor.

## OTHER USES OF MUSIC

Certain functional activities, such as crawling, stair climbing, alternate sitting and standing, can be carried out rhythmically to music with considerable advantage. In gait training and walking re-education music can also be used, either as a background to the activity or to emphasize certain aspects of the walking pattern, e.g. heel strike, push off from rear foot, and spacing of stride.

## SPECIMEN TABLES

### 1. General Warming-up Table in Standing

*Music:* 'Eye Level' (Simon Park)—single disc  
*Playing time:* 2 min 18 sec.

| | *Suggested repetitions* |
|---|---|
| 1. Stride-standing; alternate Shoulder raising and depressing. | 16 |
| 2. Stride-standing; alternate Arm punching forwards. | 8 |
| 3. Stride-standing; Trunk bending loosely from side to side. | 8 |
| 4. Standing; alternate high Knee raising. | 8 |
| 5. Standing; Heel raising. | 8 |
| 6. Stride-standing; Head turning from side to side. | 8 |
| 7. Stride-standing; Shoulder-girdle circling with emphasis on backward movement. | 12 |
| 8. Stride-standing; alternate Arm punching with Trunk turning from side to side. | 8 |
| 9. Stride-standing; rhythmical Trunk bending from side to side with alternate Arm swinging sideways-upwards over the head. | 8 |
| 10. Standing; assuming Squat position (90° bend at knees). | 8 |
| 11. Stride-standing; Head bending from side to side. | 8 |
| 12. Bend (fingers resting on chest) stride-standing; wide Elbow circling with emphasis on backward movement. | 8 |
| 13. Fist bend stride-standing; Trunk bending sideways (to left) with Arm stretching, and return to starting position, and repeat to right. | 8 |
| 14. Standing; rhythmical lunging forwards: (*a*) left Leg forwards, (*b*) right Leg forwards | 12 |

### 2. General Warming-up Table in Sitting for Chronic Chest Conditions

The exercises are arranged for use in the treatment of ambulatory patients suffering from such conditions as bronchitis, emphysema and bronchiectasis.

The patients use chairs without arms or gymnasium stools which allow a sound sitting posture.

*Music:* 'Rags and Tatters' (Geoff Love)—section of LP.  
*Playing time:* 2 min 52 sec.

|  | *Suggested repetitions* |
|---|---|
| 1. Sitting; Head bending fowards and backwards. | 8 |
| 2. Sitting; Shoulder raising and dropping ('flopping'). | 8 |
| 3. Sitting (hands resting on sides of lower ribs); emphasizing expiratory movements of chest with pressure from hands. | 8 |
| 4. Stride sitting; Trunk turning from side to side with loose Arm swinging. | 8 |
| 5. Sitting; alternate Foot tapping on floor (marching in sitting). | 16 |
| 6. Sitting; Head circling. | 8 |
| 7. Sitting; Shoulder girdle rounding and bracing. | 8 |
| 8. Sitting; rhythmical self-percussion of chest with cupped hands. | 16 |
| 9. Stride sitting; Trunk rolling. | 8 |
| 10. Sitting; Knee stretching and bending. | 8 |
| 11. Sitting; Head bending backwards (emphasis on movement of 'looking up'). | 8 |
| 12. Bend (fingers resting on chest) sitting; alternate Elbow circling backwards. | 8 |
| 13. Sitting; Arm raising sideways-upwards to touch the fingers overhead. | 8 |
| 14. Stride sitting; Trunk dropping loosely forwards to lax stoop position, and 'uncurling'. | 8 |
| 15. Sitting; rhythmical Leg parting (wide astride position) and returning to starting position. | 12 |

## MUSIC AND MOVEMENT FOR THE MENTALLY HANDICAPPED

For some of the mentally handicapped living in hospital or attending day centres regular sessions of music and movement and game-form activities provide an excellent method of improving physical fitness and giving a complete change of activity. The three groups that benefit particularly from these activities are the profoundly, severely and moderately handicapped.

In general, a fairly high staff/patient ratio is needed. Practical details of music and movement programmes for the mentally handicapped, together with organizational procedures, are given in the 3rd edition of *Progressive Exercise Therapy* (1975).

## REFERENCE

Colson J. H. C. (1975) *Progressive Exercise Therapy in Rehabilitation and Physical Education*, 3rd ed. Bristol, Wright.

# APPENDIX 1

# Starting positions

Two types of starting positions are used: Fundamental Positions and Derived Positions. The fundamental positions consist of standing, sitting, kneeling, lying and hanging. The derived positions are numerous and are obtained from the fundamental positions by altering the position of the arms, legs or trunk.

## FUNDAMENTAL POSITIONS

*Standing* (*st.*) The body is held erect with the chin level and the eyes looking forwards. The shoulders are down and slightly back; the arms hang easily by the sides with palms of the hands facing the outer sides of the thighs: fingers relaxed. The knees are straight and the feet point straight forwards, with heels and inner borders slightly apart. An alternative position for the legs (not so functionally sound) consists of having the heels together and on the same line with the toes pointing slightly outwards. The angle between the feet should not exceed 45°.

There should be no suggestion of strain or rigidity about the position.

*Sitting* (*sitt.*) The position is taken on a gymnasium stool or chair. The height, and width of seat, should allow the thighs to be fully supported, with the hips and knees flexed to 90°. The knees are slightly apart and the feet rest on the floor, toes facing forwards. The rest of the body should be held as in standing.

*Kneeling* (*kn.*) As standing, but the body-weight is supported on the knees, which are slightly apart (to increase the size of the base) or together. If the position is taken on the floor the lower legs are supported with the ankles plantar flexed; if taken on a thick mattress or plinth, with the feet over the edge (a more comfortable position), the ankles are in mid-position.

*Lying* (*ly.*) The body is fully supported in the supine position. The feet are together, with the toes pointing upwards, and the arms by the sides: fingers relaxed. The palms of the hands face the outer sides of the thighs. For exercise therapy the position is generally taken on a firm surface.

When lying is used as a starting position for various forms of movement the palms of the hands usually rest on the supporting surface. The head is also generally supported by a pillow when the position is used in the treatment of patients confined to bed. The exception to this is when head and neck and certain trunk exercises are performed.

*Hanging (hg.)* The body hangs from a horizontal beam or bar with the feet off the floor. The position of the hands varies with the type of hanging, but in over-grasp hanging (the most common type) they are pronated and at least shoulder-width apart. The body hangs at full length between the arms, which are straight, with the head held erect. The legs hang loosely with the feet together, ankles plantar flexed.

## POSITIONS DERIVED FROM STANDING
### a. By Altering Position of Arms

| | | |
|---|---|---|
| Wing standing | wg. st. | Hands rest on iliac crests, with fingers pointing forwards and thumbs behind. The shoulders are dropped and the elbows kept in line with the trunk. |
| Bend standing | bd. st. | Finger-tips are placed well back on shoulders, with elbow joints flexed, shoulder joints rotated laterally, and upper arms vertical and close to trunk. |
| Fist bend standing | Fist bd. st. | A similar position to the previous one, but the hands are clenched, the wrists are straight, and the arms are not kept so closely to the sides. (*Fig.* 225.) |
| Across bend standing | acr. bd. st. | Arms are held sideways at shoulder level, with elbows fully flexed, wrists and fingers straight, and palms facing downwards. |
| Neck rest standing | N. rst. st. | Arms are held sideways in line with trunk, with shoulder joints laterally rotated and elbow joints flexed, so that fingers are placed behind the neck at junction of head and neck. Palms face forwards; tips of fingers touch each other; wrist and fingers are straight. |
| Head rest standing | H. rst. st. | Similar to previous position, but hands are placed on top of the head, with palms facing downwards. |
| Forehead rest standing | Frh. rst. st. | As neck rest, but hands are placed on forehead with the palms facing forwards. |
| Lumbar rest standing | Lmb. rst. st. | As neck rest, but shoulder joints are rotated medially and hands are placed behind lumbar spine, palms facing backwards. |
| Heave standing | hv. st. | Upper arms are held sideways at shoulder level, with elbow joints flexed to 90°; palms face inwards. |
| Arm cross standing | A. X st. | Forearms are crossed loosely in front of chest at approximately right angles to the upper arms. Hands make contact with the upper arms. *See Fig.* 56, p. 64. |

| Low arm cross standing | low A. X st. | The arms hang loosely in front of, and close to, the body with wrists crossed. |
| Drag standing | drag st. | The arms are raised backwards as far as possible, with elbow, wrist and fingers straight, and palms facing inwards. |
| Reach standing | rch. st. | The arms are held parallel with each other in front of the body at shoulder level, with palms facing each other. The elbows, wrists and fingers are straight, and the shoulders kept down. (*Fig. 226.*) |
| Low reach standing | low rch. st. | As previous position, but the arms are held midway between reach position and the normal position by the sides of the body. |
| High reach standing | high rch. st. | As reach position, but the arms are held midway between reach and stretch positions. |
| Forearm reach standing | Forearm rch. st. | The elbow joints are flexed to 90°, with palms facing each other. (*Fig. 227.*) |
| Yard standing | yd. st. | The arms are held sideways at shoulder level, with palms facing downwards. The elbows, wrists and fingers are straight. (*Fig. 228.*) |
| Low yard standing | low yd. st. | As previous position, but arms are held midway between the yard position and the normal position by the sides of the body. |
| High yard standing | high yd. st. | As yard position, but the arms are held midway between yard and stretch positions. |
| Stretch standing | str. st. | The arms, shoulder-width apart, are stretched vertically above the head with palms facing each other. (*Fig. 229.*) |

| Fig. 225. | Fig. 226. | Fig. 227. | Fig. 228. | Fig. 229. |

## Modification of Hand Position

One or both hands may be used to grasp apparatus, so as to fix the shoulders and upper part of the body, or to give assistance to leg movements in which the body is lowered and raised, e.g. (*a*) *Low grasp sitting (chair)*; *Head bending from side to side*, and (*b*) *Low reach grasp standing (wall bars)*; *Heel raising and Knee bending*.

When one arm is employed the prefix 'half' is placed before the arm position, e.g. *Half yard grasp*. The free arm is often placed in some suitable position, e.g. *Half wing half yard grasp standing (wall bars)*; *Heel raising*.

In addition to the previous modifications arm positions may be modified further by (*a*) Changing the position of the palms, e.g. *Yard (palms forward) standing*; (*b*) Relaxing the arms, e.g. *Lax yard standing*, and (*c*) Joining the hands, e.g. *Stretch clasp standing*.

## b. By Altering Position of Trunk

| | | |
|---|---|---|
| Stoop standing | stp. st. | The trunk is inclined forwards from the hip joints with the spine kept straight. The movement is generally taken as far as the length of the hamstring muscles allows. The hips are inclined backwards by plantar flexion at ankle joints, so that balance of body is maintained. |
| Lax stoop standing | lax stp. st. | The spine and hip joints are flexed in a completely relaxed manner. The arms hang loosely downwards, and the hips are inclined backwards as in stoop standing. |
| Lax stoop back lean standing | lax stp. B. lean st. | As previous position, but with heels about 30–38 cm in front of a wall or wall bar upright, and the coccyx region in contact with it. The position is used for trunk uncurling 'vertebra by vertebra'. *See Fig.* 82, p. 82. |

## c. By Altering Position of Legs

| | | |
|---|---|---|
| Half standing | $\frac{1}{2}$ st. | Standing with the weight of the body on one leg. The other leg is either free or supported by apparatus, e.g. *Foot support side towards standing (wall bars)*. |
| Balance standing | bal. st. | Standing on beam or rib of balance bench with one foot behind the other, body facing lengthwise. (*Fig.* 230.) |
| Balance half standing | bal. $\frac{1}{2}$ st. | As previous position, but standing on one leg. The foot of the free leg hangs down by the side of the beam or rib. (*Fig.* 231.) |
| Balance across standing | bal. acr. st. | Standing on beam or rib of balance bench with feet close together and at right angles to supporting surface. (*Fig.* 232.) |
| Close standing | cl. st. | Standing with the feet pointing forwards and inner borders touching. |
| Stride standing | std. st. | Standing with feet astride, a distance of 2 foot-lengths between heels. The feet point outwards at an angle, due to the lateral rotation associated with abduction of the hip joints. |
| Wide stride standing | wd. std. st. | As previous position, but a distance of 3 foot-lengths between heels. |
| Walk forwards standing | wlk. f. st. | One leg is moved directly forwards, so that there is a distance of 2 foot-lengths between the heels. See Fig. 172, p. 143. |
| Toe standing | Toe st. | Standing on the toes, with ankle joints plantar flexed. |

| Knee bend standing (squat) | K. bd. st. | Standing on the toes with ankle joints plantar flexed and knees flexed to 90 . If feet are pointed forwards in standing position the knees are carried straight forwards over toes. If heels are together and feet pointed outwards in starting position the knees are turned outwards over the toes. |
| Knee full bend standing (full squat) | K. full bd. st. | As previous position, but knees are fully flexed. (*Fig.* 233.) |
| Instep support standing | Ins. sup. st. | Standing on one leg with dorsal surface of foot of other leg supported on stool, so that the knee joint is flexed to about 90 . The thigh is usually carried a little behind the body. The position is used for single knee bending exercises. (*Fig.* 234.) |
| Fixed standing | fix. st. | Standing with the body either facing wall bars or sideways on to the bars, with one leg raised so that the foot is fixed between the bars, with ankle joint dorsiflexed, so that the foot acts as a hook. The knee joint of fixed leg is kept extended (*Fig.* 235). |

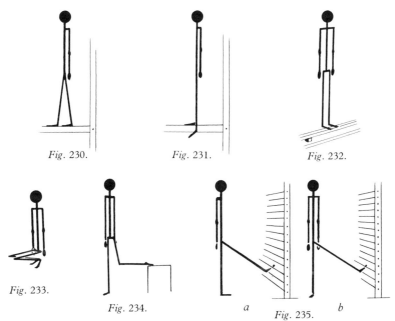

*Fig.* 230.    *Fig.* 231.    *Fig.* 232.

*Fig.* 233.

*Fig.* 234.

*a*    *Fig.* 235.    *b*

| Foot support standing | F. sup. st. | As previous position, but foot of raised leg is supported on a wall bar or the top of a balance bench. |

| Thigh support standing | Thigh sup. st. | One or both thighs are supported by the beam, which is usually placed midway between the knee and hip joints. Both thighs are supported if the patient faces the apparatus; one thigh is supported if he is sideways on to the apparatus. *See Fig.* 113, p. 94. |
|---|---|---|

## d. By Altering Position of Trunk and Legs

| Fallout forwards standing | fallout f. st. | One leg is moved forwards to a distance of about 3 foot-lengths, and the knee is bent to about 90° over the toes. The rear leg is straight and the trunk is inclined forwards in line with it. Foot of straight leg is kept in contact with floor. *See Fig.* 77, p. 77. *N.B.* The position may be taken with the thigh and buttock of forward leg supported across a gymnasium stool (fallout sitting). The toes of the rear foot rest on floor, with ankle joint plantar flexed. |
|---|---|---|
| Fallout outwards (or sideways) standing | fallout o. (or s.) st. | As previous position but the foot of the forward leg is either moved obliquely forwards-outwards or directly sideways. |

*Lunging.* When the trunk is kept erect in fallout positions it is usual to employ the term 'lunge', e.g. lunge forwards standing. It should be noted that in some gymnastic textbooks 'lunge' is used instead of 'fallout', which can be confusing.

## POSITIONS DERIVED FROM SITTING

### a. By Altering Position of Arms

As in standing.

### b. By Altering Position of Legs

| Stride sitting | std. sitt. | The feet and knees are placed apart, so that there is a distance of about 1 foot-length between the heels. The knees are flexed to 90° and the feet point obliquely outwards in line with the legs. |
|---|---|---|
| Half sitting | ½ sitt. | Sitting on apparatus, such as a plinth or high bench, with the buttock and thigh of one leg supported; the other leg is free. The position is used to allow a patient with a fixed or stiff hip joint to sit reasonably comfortably. He takes weight on his sound side and places the free limb in whatever posture is required to compensate for the fixed position of the hip. |
| Ride sitting | ride sitt. | Sitting astride apparatus, such as a chair or balance bench. The legs grip the apparatus if a very steady position is required. |

| | | |
|---|---|---|
| High ride sitting | high ride sitt. | As previous position, but taken on a high plinth; the thighs are usually strapped down. |
| Crook sitting | crk sitt. | Sitting on the floor with knees flexed to about 90°, and the soles of the feet resting on the floor. The knees may be together, without actually touching, or slightly apart. *See Fig.* 48, p. 61. |
| Cross sitting | X sitt. | Similar to crook sitting, but ankles are crossed and hips abducted and laterally rotated, so that outer aspect of each knee approaches the floor. *See Fig.* 49, p. 61. |
| Long sitting | lg. sitt. | Sitting on the floor with the legs straight, fully supported, and the same distance apart as in standing. The trunk is held erect, with hip joints flexed to about 90°, and ankle joints plantar flexed to a comfortable degree. |
| Inclined long sitting | incl. lg. sitt. | The long sitting position is taken on apparatus, such as a balance bench or stool, with heels resting on the floor. |
| Long sitting (Trunk inclined backwards with Hand support) | lg. sitt. (T. incl. b. w. Hnd. sup.) | A widely used position for certain types of leg exercises, e.g. *Quadriceps contractions* and *single Leg raising*. Seldom described in textbooks of gymnastics, probably because of the lengthy description. *See Fig.* 32*a*, p. 48. |
| Side sitting | S. sitt. | Sitting on the floor on the left or right side, with both legs bent and turned in the opposite direction. The weight of the body rests chiefly on the hip which is nearer the floor. The arm of the same side is vertical and supports the trunk. |

## c. By Altering Position of Trunk

| | | |
|---|---|---|
| Stoop sitting | stp. sitt. | As stoop standing, but the trunk movement is limited by the apposition of the thighs and abdomen. |
| Lax stoop sitting | lax stp. sitt. | As lax stoop standing. (*Fig.* 236 shows lax stoop stride sitting.) |

*Fig.* 236.

## POSITIONS DERIVED FROM KNEELING

## a. By Altering Position of Arms

As in standing.

## b. By Altering Position of Legs

| | | |
|---|---|---|
| Stride kneeling | std. kn. | The knees and feet are placed about a foot-length apart. |
| Kneel sitting | kn. sitt. | Sitting back on the heels with the trunk held erect. If a thick mattress or mat is available the position may be taken on it with the feet over the edge; this relieves the pressure on the feet and makes the position more comfortable. |
| Half kneeling | ½ kn. | Kneeling on one knee with the other leg in front of the body with the foot on the floor. Hip, knee and ankle joints of forward leg are bent to 90°. |
| Leg stretch half kneeling | L. str. ½ kn. | Kneeling on one knee with the other leg stretched in a named direction. Thus: (a) *Leg sideways stretch half kneeling.* (b) *Leg forwards stretch half kneeling.* |

## c. By Altering Position of Trunk

| | | |
|---|---|---|
| Prone kneeling | pr. kn. | The trunk is horizontal and supported by the arms and thighs, which are vertical. The hip and knee joints are flexed to 90°. The correct position of spine and head is maintained. (*Fig.* 237.) |

*Fig.* 237.

## POSITIONS DERIVED FROM LYING

### a. By Altering Position of Arms

As in standing.

### b. By Altering Position of Legs

| | | |
|---|---|---|
| Crook lying | cr. ly. | Lying with the soles of the feet resting on the floor. The knees are flexed to varying degrees, but the usual position is about 90°. |
| Stride crook lying | std. cr. ly. | As previous position, but the legs and feet are placed astride, with the heels about 45 cm apart. The feet point obliquely outwards in line with the legs. |
| Crook lying with Pelvis raised | cr. ly. w. P. rais. | From crook lying position the pelvis is raised until there is a straight line between the trunk and the thighs. |

| | | |
|---|---|---|
| Leg lift lying | L. lift ly. | Lying with the legs raised; the range of movement must be indicated, e.g. *Vertical leg lift lying*. The legs are kept together, with the knees extended and the ankles plantar flexed. |
| Stride lying | std. ly. | Lying with feet astride as in stride standing. |
| Half lying | $\frac{1}{2}$ ly. | Lying on a plinth or bed with the trunk supported by a back rest or pillows in a position midway between lying and sitting upright. The legs are straight and fully supported. |
| Crook half lying | crk. $\frac{1}{2}$ ly. | As half lying, but the knees are flexed and the feet rest on the plinth or bed as in crook lying. |
| Prone lying | pr. ly. | Lying face downwards with the body fully supported. This is an unpleasant position for the face, and so the head is generally turned to one side. Similarly, the arms are often allowed to rest on the supporting surface with the palms turned upwards instead of being held to the sides as in lying. |
| Leg prone lying | L. pr. ly. | Lying face down on a high plinth, or plinth, in such a manner that only the legs are supported (from the iliac crests downwards), and the trunk lies unsupported in the horizontal plane. The ankles are strapped down to the plinth. The chin is kept in and the arms are by the sides, as in the lying position. A stool is placed under the trunk, so that the hands can rest on it and support the trunk during rest periods. |
| Fixed high Thigh support across prone lying | fix. high Th. sup. acr. pr. ly. | As prone lying, but the thighs rest across apparatus, such as a stool, or two balance benches placed one on top of the other. The feet are fixed by the wall bars or living support. The trunk, head and legs form a straight line with the chin kept in. The arms are by the sides, as in lying. (*Fig.* 238.) Strong extension exercises for the spine and hips are given from this position. |
| Side-lying | S.-ly. | Lying on one side. The under arm is either allowed to rest loosely in front of the body, or is bent up, so that the hand supports the head. As the position is unstable, the under leg is sometimes placed a little in front of the other one. Alternatively, the under leg is flexed at the hip and knee joints. |

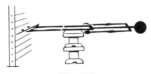

*Fig.* 238.

## POSITIONS DERIVED FROM HANGING

### By Altering Position of Legs

| | | |
|---|---|---|
| Angle hanging | ang. hg. | Hanging with the feet resting on the floor. The hips are flexed, the knees extended and the ankles plantar flexed. The arms are straight and shoulder-width apart. (*Fig. 239.*) |
| Fall hanging | fall hg. | Hanging from the beam with the body obliquely forward, and the feet or heels resting on the floor. The legs and trunk should be in a straight line. The arms are generally described as being 'vertical'. In practice, however, when the position is used for arm bending exercises it is better to have the arms at right angles to the trunk. Over-grasp position for the hands is used. (*Fig. 240.*) |
| Horizontal fall hanging | hor. fall hg. | As fall hanging, but the feet rest on apparatus, such as a stool, or the ankles are held by living support. In the latter case the legs are parted, the supporter holding the ankles in the same way as the handles of a wheelbarrow. |
| Reverse hanging | rev. hg. | Hanging with the head downwards. The position is generally taken on the wall bars. |

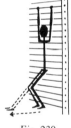

*Fig.* 239.

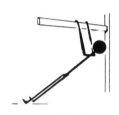

*Fig.* 240.

### Grasp Positions used in Hanging

| | | |
|---|---|---|
| Over grasp | over gr. | Grasping apparatus with hands in pronated position. |
| Under grasp | und. gr. | Grasping apparatus with hands in supinated position. |
| Alternate grasp | alt. gr. | Grasping apparatus with one hand supinated and the other pronated. |
| Inward grasp | inw. gr. | Grasping apparatus with the palms facing inwards. |

*N.B.* When the wall bars are used for hanging positions, it is usual to omit any reference to the grasp. *Hanging (wall bars)* indicates that the position is taken with the back towards the bars. *Towards hanging (wall bars)* is used when the body faces the bars.

## OTHER DERIVED POSITIONS

| | | |
|---|---|---|
| Prone falling | pr. fall. | The body, which is in a straight line from head to heels (and faces the floor), rests on the hands and toes. The arms are vertical and shoulder-width apart, with elbows extended. Hands are generally turned inwards. (*Fig.* 241.) |
| Inclined prone falling | incl. pr. fall. | As previous position, but the hands are supported on apparatus: beam, wall bars or stool. (*Fig.* 242.) |
| Horizontal prone falling | hor. pr. fall. | As prone falling, but the feet are supported on the beam or a stool, so that the body is in the horizontal position. *See Fig.* 66, p. 72. |
| Side falling | S. fall. | The body, kept straight, and with one side turned towards the floor, rests on one hand and one foot. The supporting arm is vertical with elbow extended. *See Fig.* 111, p. 93. |
| Inclined side falling | incl. s. fall. | As previous position, but the supporting hand rests on the beam or a stool. |
| Horizontal side falling | hor. S. fall. | As side falling, but the feet are supported on the beam or a stool, so that the body is in the horizontal position. *See Fig.* 115, p. 94. |
| Horizontal half standing | hor. $\frac{1}{2}$ st. | Standing on one leg with the body and the free leg in the horizontal plane. Free leg is kept straight, in line with the trunk, with ankle joint plantar flexed. N.B. An arched position may be assumed. |
| Balance hanging | bal. hg. | The body, facing forwards and supported by hands and thighs, rests across the beam. The body is arched and held as near to the horizontal as possible; the legs are pressed lightly backwards. The arms are straight and parallel. (*Fig.* 243.) |
| Front rest | fr. rst. | A similar position to balance hanging, but the body is held in a straight line and the forward leaning is restricted to about 15°. Apparatus such as the beam, or beam saddle on beam, may be used. (*Fig.* 244.) |

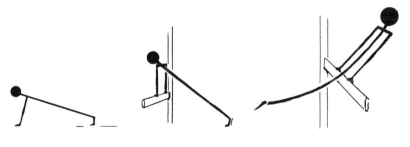

*Fig.* 241.          *Fig.* 242.          *Fig.* 243.

Crouch
sitting

crch. sitt.

The body is supported by the toes and hands, which rest on the floor, with hips and knees flexed as much as possible, and trunk inclined forwards. The arms are vertical and may be outside the thighs (close crouch) or between the thighs (open crouch). (*Fig.* 245.)

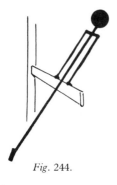

*Fig.* 244.

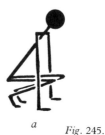

*a*

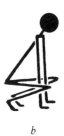

*b*

*Fig.* 245.

# APPENDIX 2

# Gymnastic terminology

Throughout this book the terminology used to describe the exercises and gymnastic movements is based on that standardized some years ago by the Ling Physical Education Association.* The method of description and technical terms used, with some additions and modifications, are given in full in this appendix, along with the various abbreviations used to facilitate the writing of exercise programmes.

Gymnastic terminology, being largely descriptive in character, is particularly suitable for describing the specific forms of movement used in exercise therapy. It is sometimes criticized, however, as being cumbersome and complicated. On the other hand, it must be emphasized that other systems of recording movement in use today are infinitely more complicated and difficult to learn. Benesh Movement Notation, for example, is based on an elaborate system of signs which are written on a five-line stave within a square or frame. Laban Notation (widely used in movement studies) is also based on a system of signs.

## TERMS DENOTING MOVEMENT

| | | |
|---|---|---|
| Bending | bend. | Flexion of the part indicated. N.B. Extension of the spine from the neutral position is referred to as 'bending backwards', e.g. *Fixed prone lying; Trunk bending backwards with Arm turning outwards.* |
| Bracing | brac. | The term indicates either the stabilization of a joint or the drawing together of two parts. It is used mainly in connection with hyperextension of the knee and adduction of the scapulae, e.g. (*a*) *Standing; Heel raising and Knee bracing,* (*b*) *Sitting; Shoulder bracing.* |
| Carrying | carry. | The arm(s) or leg(s) is moved in a horizontal direction. |
| Circling (on apparatus) | circl. | Circling over or under apparatus, such as the beam, from which the body is suspended by the hands. |

---

*Now the Physical Education Association of Gt. Britain and N. Ireland.

| Circling or rolling | circl. or roll. | The part of the body indicated is moved smoothly in a circular direction. N.B. In *rolling in rings* the body as a whole is moved, the toes acting as the fixed point. |
| Closing | clos. | The arm(s) or leg(s) is moved towards the midline of the body. |
| Flinging | fling. | A quick elbow extension from the across-bend position. |
| Lowering | lower. | The part of the body indicated is lowered in a straight line from its axis of movement. |
| Raising or lifting | raise. or lift. | The part of the body indicated is raised in a straight line from its axis of movement. |
| Rebound | reb. | A term used in connection with rhythmical jumping and hopping. It indicates that a second, subsidiary jump follows the first main jump. |
| Recoil | recoil | A controlled slackening off of a muscle group after a position has been reached, e.g. *Forearm reach (lax fingers) sitting; strong Finger bending and slow recoil.* |
| Tilting | tilt. | A term used in connection with forward-backward movement of the pelvis on the femoral heads. Lateral tilting of the pelvis is usually described as 'hip updrawing'. |

# TERMS DENOTING TYPE OF MOVEMENT

| Single | 1 | The term is used when one arm (or leg) is moved *in turn* with the other arm (or leg), or when one arm (or leg) is moved *several times* in succession before the other arm (or leg) is exercised, e.g. (a) *Standing; single Arm raising forwards,* (b) *Forearm reach sitting; single Forearm turning inwards and outwards continuously to a given count.* *Single* is also used when one limb only is to be exercised; the term is then qualified by additional information, e.g. *Reach grasp high half standing (beam and block); single (affected) Leg swinging forwards and backwards.* |
| Alternate | alt. | The term is used when one arm (or leg) moves towards one limit of the movement while the other arm (or leg) moves towards the other limit, e.g. *Walk forwards standing; alternate Arm swinging forwards and backwards.* |

## TERMS DENOTING DIRECTION OF MOVEMENT

| | | | | | |
|---|---|---|---|---|---|
| Across | acr. | Inclined | incl. | Outwards | o. |
| Backwards | b. | Inwards | inw. | Right | r. |
| Behind | beh. | Lateral | lat. | Sideways | s. |
| Downwards | d. | Left | l. | Under | und. |
| Forwards | f. | Medial | med. | Upwards | u. |
| Horizontal | hor. | Oblique | obl. | | |

## TERMS INDICATING POSITION OF LIMBS AND TRUNK

| | | | | | |
|---|---|---|---|---|---|
| Bend | bd. | Kneeling | kn. | Squatting | squat. |
| Close | cl. | Long | lg. | Standing | st. |
| Crook | crk. | Lying | ly. | Stretch | str. |
| Cross | X | Prone | pr. | Stride | std. |
| Crouch | crch. | Reach | rch. | Wing | wg. |
| Grasp | gr. | Relaxed | lax. | Yard | yd. |
| Hanging | hg. | Rest | rst. | | |
| Heave | hv. | Sitting | sitt. | | |

*N.B.* In abbreviating terms used to describe movement, rather than position, which end in -ing (bending, stretching, carrying, etc.) the final syllable is omitted. *See* Terms denoting Movement, p. 273.

## PARTS OF THE BODY AND THEIR ABBREVIATIONS

| | | | | | |
|---|---|---|---|---|---|
| Abdomen | Abd. | Hand(s) | Hnd. | Pelvis | P. |
| Ankle(s) | Ank. | Head | H. | Shoulder(s) | Sh. |
| Arm(s) | A. | Heel(s) | Hl. | Shoulder | Sh. bl. |
| Back | B. | Hip(s) | Hp. | blades | |
| Chest | Ch. | Instep | Ins. | Side | S. |
| Elbow(s) | Elb. | Knee(s) | K. | Thigh(s) | Th. |
| Feet | F. | Leg(s) | L. | Toe(s) | Toe |
| Finger(s) | Fing. | Neck | N. | Trunk | T. |
| Forehead | Frh. | Palm(s) | Pa. | Wrist(s) | Wr. |

## TERMS REFERRING TO THE POSITION OF THE BODY IN RELATION TO APPARATUS OR LIVING SUPPORT

| | | |
|---|---|---|
| Fixed | fix. | One or both feet are fixed in or under apparatus, such as wall bars, or by a partner. |
| High | high | The term is used to indicate that a position is taken on apparatus (e.g. *high sitting*); it may also be employed in exercises to indicate that a movement is to be taken as far as possible, e.g. *Lying; high Knee raising.* The term is also used to modify such positions as yard and reach, e.g. *high yard.* |
| Support | sup. | The part of the body named is supported by apparatus. |
| Living support | (.) | A partner provides support, e.g. *Over-grasp horizontal fall hanging (beam and living support); Arm bending.* (..) represents two supporters. |

| Towards | tow. | The body faces apparatus. When grasp positions are used it is not necessary to use the term. |
| Back towards | B. tow. | The back is turned towards the apparatus. When the hanging position is taken at the wall bars with the back towards the bars, it is usual to dispense with the term 'back towards'. |
| Side towards | S. tow. | One side of the body is turned towards the apparatus. When a grasp position is used it is not customary to use the term. |

## METHOD OF DESCRIBING EXERCISES IN TERMINOLOGY

1. The name of the starting position is given first; it is followed by a description of the movement to be performed. A semi-colon is used to separate the starting position from the movement, e.g. *Lying; high Knee raising.*

2. The term *half* ($\frac{1}{2}$) is used to prefix the starting position when one limb only is involved, e.g. *Half yard grasp standing (wall bars).*

3. In describing the movement, the part of the body moved is mentioned first, and then the type and direction of the movement. When more than one part of the body is involved the following order is usually suggested: Head, Arms, Trunk, Legs, Feet. This sequence is modified, however, when describing exercises where the movement of one part of the body is more important than the other subsidiary movements involved. This part is mentioned first, e.g. (*a*) *Fixed prone lying; Trunk bending backwards with Arm turning outwards and single Leg raising backwards and (b) Standing; Heel raising and Knee full bending with loose Arm swinging forwards-backwards.*

It is unnecessary to mention the return movement unless it is intended that the return movement shall not be the opposite of the original movement.

4. In describing movements of the limbs the plural is indicated by Arm (A.), Leg (L.), Knee (K.) etc. When one limb is to be moved on its own, or in turn with the other limb, the term *single* (1) is used. *See* Terms denoting type of Movement, p. 274.

5. When a movement consists of several parts a comma is used to separate each part, e.g. *Prone kneeling; single high Knee raising, Leg stretching and raising backwards, and return to starting position.* Brackets are used to give information concerning the method of performing the exercise (including counts and beats), type of apparatus and support used, e.g. *Towards standing (balance bench); stepping up forwards, affected Leg leading (1–2), and stepping down backwards, affected Leg leading (3–4).*

6. In abbreviating terminology a full stop is used after each abbreviation employed, e.g.

(*a*) *pr. kn.; P. tilt. f. and b. w. H. bend. b. and f.*
(*b*) *st.; Hl. rais. w. A. swing. f. and f.-u.*
(*c*) *N. rst. fix. pr. ly.; T. bend. b. w. turn.*

## REFERENCES

Laban R. (1975) *Modern Educational Dance*. Plymouth, Macdonald & Evans.
Ling Physical Education Association (1950) *Terminology of Swedish Educational Gymnastics*. London.
McGuiness-Scott J. (1980) Benesh Movement Notation: an introduction to recording clinical data. *Physiotherapy* **66**, 268–270.

# Bibliography

### General Surgery

Aird I. (1957) *A Companion in Surgical Studies*, 2nd ed. Edinburgh, Livingstone.
Ballinger W. F. and Drapanas T. (1972) *Practice of Surgery*. St Louis, Mosby.
Bendixen H. H. (1965) *Respiratory Care*. St Louis, Mosby.
Macfarlane D. A. and Thomas L. P. (1977) *Textbook of Surgery*, 4th ed. Edinburgh, Churchill Livingstone.

### Orthopaedic Surgery

Adams J. C. (1980) *Standard Orthopaedic Operations*, 2nd ed. Edinburgh, Churchill Livingstone.
Charnley J. (1970) Total hip replacement by low friction arthroplasty. *Clin. Orthop.* **72**, 7.
Duthrie R. B. and Ferguson A. B. (1973) *Mercer's Orthopaedic Surgery*, 7th ed. Edinburgh, Churchill Livingstone.
Edmonson A. S. and Crenshaw A. H. (ed.) (1980) *Campbell's Operative Orthopaedics*, Vol. 2, 6th ed. St Louis, Mosby.
Longton E. B. (1973) Orthopaedic surgery in arthritic lower limb joints. *Physiotherapy* **59**, 116–119.
Muller M. E. (1970) Total hip prosthesis. *Clin. Orthop.* **72**, 46.
Smillie I. S. (1978) *Injuries of the Knee Joint*, 5th ed. Edinburgh, Churchill Livingstone.

### Physical Education

Knudsen K. A. (1947) *Textbook of Gymnastics*, 2nd ed. London, Churchill.
Laban R. (1975) *Modern Educational Dance*. Plymouth, Macdonald & Evans.
Laban R. and Lawrence A. (1974) *Effort*. Plymouth, Macdonald & Evans.
Larson L. A. (1974). *Fitness, Health, and Work Capacity*. New York, Macmillan.
Ling Physical Education Association (1950) *Terminology of Swedish Educational Gymnastics*. London.
Mace R. and Benn B. (1982) *Gymnastic Skills*. London, Batsford.
Morgan R. E. and Adamson G. T. (1961) *Circuit Training*, 2nd ed. London, Bell.
Munrow A. D. (1963) *Pure and Applied Gymnastics*, 2nd ed. London, Arnold.
Thulin J. G. (1947) *Gymnastic Handbook*. Lund, South Swedish Gymnastic Institute.
Verducci F. M. (1980) *Measurement Concepts in Physical Education*. St. Louis, Mosby.

## Physical Treatment

American College of Sports Medicine (1980) *Guide Lines for Graded Exercise Testing and Exercise Prescription*, 2nd ed. Philadelphia, Lea & Febiger.

Basmajian J. V. (ed.) (1980) *Therapeutic Exercise*. Baltimore, Williams & Wilkins.

Butler P. and Kepson G. (1980) Quadriceps strengthening: a comparative study of three types of apparatus for strengthening the quadriceps femoris muscle dynamically. *Physiotherapy* 66, 82–85.

DeLorme T. L. (1945) Restoration of muscle power by heavy resistance exercises. *J. Bone Joint Surg.* 27, 646–667.

DeLorme T. L. and Watkins A. L. (1945) Technics of progressive resistance exercises. *Arch. Phys. Med.* 29, 263–273.

DeLorme T. L. and Watkins A. L. (1951) *Progressive Resistance Exercises: Technique and Medical Application*. New York, Appleton-Century-Crofts.

Dick F. W. (1968) A review of recent studies pertaining to strength. *Br. J. Sports Med.* 4, 35–41.

Edwards R. H. T. and McDonnell M. (1974) Handheld dynamometer for evaluating voluntary muscle function. *Lancet* 2, 757.

Gardiner D. M. (1981) *The Principles of Exercise Therapy*, 4th ed. London, Bell & Hyman.

Hale G. (ed.) (1979) *The Source Book for the Disabled*. New York, Paddington Press.

Hollis M. (1981) *Practical Exercise Therapy*, 2nd ed. Oxford, Blackwell Scientific Publications.

Hirschberg G. G., Lewis L. and Vaughan P. (1976) *Rehabilitation*, 2nd ed. Philadelphia, Lippincott.

McQueen I. (1954) Recent advances in the techniques of progressive resistance exercises. *Br. Med. J.* 2, 1193–1198.

Nicoll E. A. (1941) Rehabilitation of the injured. *Br. Med. J.* 1, 501–506.

Nicoll E. A. (1943) Principles of exercise therapy. *Br. Med. J.* 1, 747–750.

Smith Guthrie O. F. (1943) *Rehabilitation, Re-education and Remedial Exercises*. London, Baillière, Tindall & Cox.

Vannier M. (1977) *Physical Activities for the Handicapped*. New Jersey, Prentice-Hall.

Wells K. F. and Luttgens K. (1982) *Kinesiology*, 7th ed. Philadelphia, Saunders College Publishers.

Westers B. M. (1982) Factors influencing strength testing and exercise prescription. *Physiotherapy* 68, 42–44.

Wynn Parry C. B. (1973) *Rehabilitation of the Hand*, 3rd ed. London, Butterworths.

Zinovieff A. (1951) Heavy resistance exercises: the Oxford Technique. *Br. J. Phys. Med. Indust. Hyg.* 14, 129.

## Anatomy and Physiology

Green J. H. (1975) *Basic Clinical Physiology*, 2nd ed. London, Oxford University Press.

Guyton A. (1979) *Physiology of the Human Body*, 5th ed. Philadelphia, Saunders.

McMinn R. M. H. and Hutchings R. T. (1978) *A Colour Atlas of Human Anatomy*. London, Wolfe Medical.

Williams P. L. and Warwick R. (1980) *Gray's Anatomy*, 36th ed. Edinburgh, Churchill Livingstone.

# INDEX